THE
PREGNANT
ATHLETE

THE PREGNANT ATHLETE

HOW TO STAY IN YOUR BEST SHAPE EVER—BEFORE, DURING, AND AFTER PREGNANCY

BRANDI DION, NSCA-CPT, USAT LI
STEVEN DION, EdD

WITH JOEL B. HELLER, MD, WITH PERRY McINTOSH

Da Capo
LIFE
LONG

A Member of the Perseus Books Group

Designed by Trish Wilkinson
Set in 11-point Minion Pro

Library of Congress Cataloging-in-Publication Data

Dion, Brandi.
   The pregnant athlete : how to stay in your best shape ever—before, during, and after pregnancy / Brandi Dion, NSCA-CPT, USAT LI, Steven Dion, EdD ; with Joel B. Heller, MD ; with Perry McIntosh.
      pages cm
   Includes index.
   ISBN 978-0-7382-1726-0 (pbk.) — ISBN 978-0-7382-1727-7 (e-book)
1. Exercise for pregnant women. 2. Pregnant women—Health and hygiene. 3. Physical fitness for women. I. Dion, Steven. II. Heller, Joel B. III. McIntosh, Perry. IV. Title.
   RG558.7.D66 2014
   618.2'44—dc23

                                                                   2013045525

First Da Capo Press edition 2014

Published by Da Capo Press
A Member of the Perseus Books Group
www.dacapopress.com

Note: The information in this book is true and complete to the best of our knowledge. This book is intended only as an informative guide for those wishing to know more about health issues. In no way is this book intended to replace, countermand, or conflict with the advice given to you by your own physician. The ultimate decision concerning care should be made between you and your doctor. We strongly recommend you follow his or her advice. Information in this book is general and is offered with no guarantees on the part of the authors or Da Capo Press. The authors and publisher disclaim all liability in connection with the use of this book.

Da Capo Press books are available at special discounts for bulk purchases in the United States by corporations, institutions, and other organizations. For more information, please contact the Special Markets Department at the Perseus Books Group, 2300 Chestnut Street, Suite 200, Philadelphia, PA, 19103, or call (800) 810-4145, ext. 5000, or e-mail special.markets@perseusbooks.com.

10 9 8 7 6 5 4 3 2 1

To our inspirations:
Mackenzie Spider-One Dion and Maddox Wolverine Dion

Contents

Acknowledgments

Thanks to all who helped make this book a reality. Although it was inspired by a *lack* of information and examples to keep me in top shape during my first pregnancy, help arrived early on from my ob-gyn, Dr. Joel Heller. Thanks, Dr. Heller, for the initial nudge to write this book and for contributing so much to its content! We also want to thank Perry McIntosh for all her efforts in helping us tell our story, Jenna Dudevoir for being our pregnant model, the B&S Fitness and CrossFit IronSpider community and coaches, our mothers, who help with our kids so we can live a sane lifestyle of racing and training, and of course our two energetic, challenging, life-sucking children, Mackenzie and Maddox, whom we love dearly—we couldn't have done it without them!

We must also give a shout-out to Joanne Wyckoff, our agent, and to Renee Sedliar and the talented folks at Da Capo Press for believing in our book and recognizing its value to all pregnant athletes.

Foreword

I was recently looking through my old copy of *Williams Obstetrics*, the leading reference for obstetricians. In this 1,500-page book, I found less than a single page on exercise. Yet in over twenty years of practice, I have seen more and more interest in fitness among patients—and I've seen more athletic patients, with various degrees of vocation and avocation, every year. Luckily, the American College of Obstetrics and Gynecology (ACOG) updated its guidelines on exercise during pregnancy about ten years ago. The Centers for Disease Control guidelines agree that healthy women can continue even vigorous activity through pregnancy. In fact, both these organizations encourage regular moderate exercise for *all* pregnant women. Doctors now understand that a woman's prepregnancy conditioning largely determines what is safe, and the ACOG supports intense exercise in that context as long as the woman feels good and the pregnancy remains normal. This means that a physically active woman can be frank with her physician about her level of activity, and she can work with her medical team to monitor her health and her baby's development.

One of the joys of practicing obstetrics and gynecology is discussing common interests with my patients. When Brandi and Steve Dion asked for my assistance in writing this book, I was excited and flattered. I have been caring for female athletes and active women for over twenty years, and exercise physiology has been a personal interest since college. Personally, I have always made personal fitness and competition a priority and so I try to support and encourage my patients to maintain fitness as a way of improving their quality of life and preventing disease. I have always marveled at the adaptations the body undertakes in growing and delivering a human being over a nine-month period and been happy to see patients who are motivated to continue to be very active throughout pregnancy. With care and planning, and by paying attention to the body as it changes, many women can maintain their athletic programs almost to the day of delivery. Unfortunately, there will be complicated pregnancies, where none of this will apply and activity may need to be drastically modified. In this vein, please review your activities and training with your health-care provider, as he or she knows you and can best guide you in whether an activity is safe.

Throughout this book, you'll learn about the adaptations the body makes during pregnancy and how you as an athlete can work with them to maintain fitness and strength—for your health and your baby's. In Brandi and Steve, you'll find two coaches who've been there—as the parents of two kids, they've been on both sides of the pregnant athlete experience as mom-to-be and as partner of mom-to-be. As fitness professionals, they realized that there was not a lot written to serve as guidance to pregnant athletes who wanted to maintain a high level of fitness despite receiving negative input from family or unenthusiastic health-care providers. In this book, they offer the most recent research and science, as well as personal experience to help guide any athlete committed to being active throughout her pregnancy, with explanations that make sense. Their years of experience as athletes and personal trainers allow them to challenge themselves and their clients.

I anticipate that this book will be updated one day when there is even more known about the effects of exercise on pregnancy. In traditional societies, women put their body through much stress, caring for large families and surviving while at the same time being pregnant. Evolution favors those who stay strong and subject their body to healthy amounts of physical stress, as seen by slowing of the aging process in those who stay active. This does not mean restrictions in nutrition, however, for harm does come to pregnancy in times of famine. This book emphasizes the importance of adequate calorie intake through a balanced diet, whether exercising or not.

Our goal is simple: to help you have a safe, healthy pregnancy—one where you will also feel safe and healthy engaging in your athletic pursuits. I hope that this book will inspire you to continue to be passionate about competition and fitness while at the same time creating a healthy newborn.

Joel B. Heller, MD

Introduction

With so much information available for pregnant women today, why should you turn to this book? The answer is simple: because you are serious about fitness and you are thinking about becoming pregnant or are already a mother-to-be. You want to have a safe and healthy pregnancy *and* maintain a high level of fitness. And you want to do it without sneaking your workouts in or feeling guilty. Here's the good news: You can do it! How do I know? Because I've done it—twice! My own experiences as a very pregnant athlete who raced and worked out can serve as an example of what pregnant athletes are capable of doing. The workout routines in this book are just a few of the many that I completed through my two pregnancies, keeping me challenged and inspired to race right up to delivery. In fact, I completed our local 5-mile Thanksgiving Turkey Trot ("Turkey Waddle" in my case!) four days before my son's due date. And I'm not the only woman who's successfully maintained her fitness throughout pregnancy. I've worked with other pregnant athletes—you'll be hearing from some of

them and from other women throughout this book, too.

I wasn't always so confident about training through pregnancy. I was a thirty-two-year-old triathlete and in peak condition before my first pregnancy. I had just finished my best race season ever and decided to turn my attention to starting a family. I told myself I would be happy to be pregnant and to focus on having a baby instead of racing and training. Still, scared by stories of other moms whose lives seemed transformed in ways they didn't want or expect, I worried that I would never get back into the shape that I had been in for so long. To add to my anxiety, suddenly I was walking on eggshells, because everyone had advice on what I should be doing—prenatal yoga and walking—and shouldn't be doing: running, lifting, biking, working out, and of course racing—all the things I love and live for. What was I supposed to do, just take it easy? As much as I like chocolate, I just wasn't ready to put up my feet, open a big bag of M&M's, and give up exercise for nine months! I scoured the shelves at the local bookstores, searched the Internet for anything related to "pregnant athletes," "pregnant triathletes," "strength training and pregnancy," anything that would come close to relating to my life and intensity level. Finding absolutely nothing, I became very frustrated in my search and decided just to listen to my body and be careful.

> "I know I run to stay sane. But that's also who my friends are, that's what I talk about, that's what I think about. It drove me crazy during my first pregnancy to just be online reading about it and not knowing how much I could do. By the second one I was just like, 'Screw it—I'm just going to do what I want to do.'"
>
> —MOLLY, RUNNER, MOM OF TWO

I had heard from so many people that women shouldn't train at high intensity during pregnancy that when I first got pregnant, I was ready to give up on my high-performance training and intensity because I simply didn't know any better. After I got that exciting positive test result on the pee stick I was nervous about working out at my usual level. I couldn't just stop working out, so I decided to continue my usual training but at reduced intensity until my first prenatal appointment, scheduled at twelve weeks. If you've ever tried to cut back your intensity, then you know that this is harder than it sounds. It doesn't take much to get the heart rate into the supposed "danger zone." This was the longest twelve weeks of my life!

Now, two athletic pregnancies later, I know better. I now know that if a woman has a healthy, normal pregnancy, there is no reason she should not continue with any exercise regimen that she is accustomed to following. Of course, pregnancy is not the time to up the ante or take up a new intense activity, but the American Congress of Obstetricians and Gynecologists now supports continuing exercise at accustomed levels for women with normal, healthy pregnancies.

I chose to hold on to being an athlete even as I became a mom. I wanted to continue pushing my limits, even if my limits were changing. I had always trusted my body to tell me what it could do and I didn't see any reason for pregnancy to change that. Athletes know that the mind is always ready to give up or give in before the body—so I listened to my body, and my body told me I could keep up my fitness routines.

If you are like me, this book is for you. *The Pregnant Athlete* focuses on how pregnancy affects your body, mind, and emotions as an athlete, and what you need to do to sustain your conditioning as well as keep yourself happy during those nine months and beyond. If you are serious about your sport or your passion for fitness—at a recreational or competitive level—you probably want to keep going and try your best to maintain as high a level of fitness as you can during your pregnancy even while everything becomes harder to do. Of course, you will use good common sense, but you want to do what you can for as long as you can and be confident in doing that. That attitude will keep your mind off the inevitable weight gain and discomfort and will give your experience with pregnancy a positive focus, not to mention some good laughs. Here's how we will achieve this together.

- We take a good look at how your body changes over nine months (and after!) and how those changes impact your fitness efforts. Your body is manufacturing special hormones that affect your lungs and ligaments, not to mention your moods and your appetite. And that growing baby bump will throw off your balance and make some activities all but impossible.
- Dr. Joel Heller, ob-gyn, offers advice and wisdom based on the latest research and his own practice, having worked with countless pregnant athletes (including me!)
- I share my story as a triathlete, coach, boot camp instructor, weight lifter, CrossFitter, wife, and mother: the ups and downs and lessons learned during two very active and racing pregnancies. Granted, as a fitness professional, I have more time to devote to exercise than most women do. But rest assured, I faced the same challenges you will face over the course of two pregnancies.
- You'll be hearing from other pregnant athletes, too—moms who stayed committed to their fitness routines and have lots of knowledge and support to share.

- Steve Dion (professor of health and exercise science and my husband) shares his insights as a fitness professional and as the partner of a pregnant athlete.
- Workouts with familiar moves modified to be appropriate to the different stages of pregnancy will keep you challenged, active, and strong—physically, mentally, and emotionally—for the whole year before, during, and after your pregnancy.
- As an athlete, you know that nutrition is key. We'll talk a lot about ways to fuel your pregnancy and workouts, making sure you stay healthy through all nine months and beyond.

WHY EXERCISE THROUGH PREGNANCY?

Even if you never compete, there are so many reasons to maintain your high level of fitness through your pregnancy. As an athlete, you know that exercise benefits almost everyone—pregnant or not—by increasing energy; improving mood; promoting muscle tone, strength, and endurance; and improving sleep. And pregnancy is hard work; being strong physically, mentally, and emotionally will help your body carry the baby in relative comfort. ACOG adds a few more benefits to the list for pregnant women: reducing backache, constipation, bloating, and swelling, and reducing the risk and severity of gestational diabetes. Are there any of these outcomes you *don't* want to achieve?

But wait—there's more! Studies show that women who continue endurance exercise at or near prepregnancy levels gain less weight than do those who stop exercising before the twenty-eighth week, and their babies are a healthier weight, too. Babies of exercising mothers are healthier at birth and better manage the stress of delivery. They have a lower heart rate and sleep through the night sooner than do babies of more sedentary moms. Other benefits, including higher IQ test scores later in life, are reported but not well studied yet. Still, are there any of these outcomes that you don't want to achieve?

But the most important reason to keep up your exercise is that fitness—whatever your sport—is part of who you are. So many women feel the same as my friend Meghan, a dancer, who told me, "It's what my body does and has always done. It shouldn't change because of pregnancy." Or Carol, a runner, "I don't feel that life needs to change all that much just because you are baking a baby." Pregnancy is a huge adjustment—but that doesn't mean sacrificing who you are and what's important to you.

WHAT DO I MEAN BY "EXERCISE"?

Only some kinds of exercise during your pregnancy can lead to these results. According to Dr. Joseph Clapp, who has studied exercise and its effects in pregnant women for decades, exercise should be

- Intense: You should perceive your exercise as somewhat hard (see "Before you Conceive" for an explanation of rate of perceived exertion [RPE]).
- Sustained: Aim for sessions of 30 to 90 minutes.
- Frequent: Five times a week allows two rest days, which are as important as your workouts.

> "I was thirty-six when I got pregnant. I waited so long to get pregnant because I didn't want to give up the movement that I love. Now that I know I don't have to give it up, I may decide to have another child."
> —MEGHAN, DANCER, MOTHER OF ONE

The exercises and workouts in this book build *functional* strength, designed to support you in real life, in real situations. They will help build and maintain your strength for what is potentially going to be the most athletic event of your life—childbirth. If you stop training, you are not helping your body or your baby prepare for delivery. During both pregnancies, my workouts were constantly varied, high intensity, and built on a lot of mini sets. My goal in sharing them in each chapter is to demonstrate what I was able to do in that month. I hope they motivate you to do what *you* can. Everyone has different interests and needs, and no one program will meet them all. You can follow my workouts as I did them, or use the templates we provide to customize workouts based on your own training and exercise goals and ambitions. A solid program is constructed in a manner that addresses the major areas of fitness, and this is exactly what we have put together for you.

WHEN SHOULD YOU NOT EXERCISE?

The generally accepted rule of thumb is that you should be able to exercise at your prepregnancy levels *if you have a normal, healthy pregnancy.* ACOG considers the following conditions to be "absolute contraindications" to aerobic exercise during pregnancy:

- Significant heart or lung disease
- Incompetent cervix
- Multiple gestation at risk for premature labor
- Persistent second or third trimester bleeding
- Placenta previa after twenty-six weeks
- Premature labor during this pregnancy
- Ruptured membranes
- Pregnancy-induced hypertension

And remember that pregnancy is a long process and, unfortunately, events or a change in your health can move your pregnancy out of the "normal, healthy" category and into a situation where more care and watchful attention are needed. The cause may be unrelated to your exercise program, but it may well affect your ability to continue.

Stop exercising and see your doctor if any of these warning signs occur:

- Vaginal bleeding
- Prolonged dizziness or faintness
- Chest pain
- Persistent headache or out-of-the-ordinary muscle weakness
- Calf swelling or pain
- Uterine contractions
- Big decrease in fetal movement
- Fluid leaking from the vagina

These developments are rare, and it's most likely you'll have smooth sailing through all nine months. Always follow the advice of your medical practitioner and put the health and safety of your baby first. Keep in mind that pregnancy is temporary. Even though we all want to maintain our fitness routine, it will not be the end of the world (as much as it might seem like it!) to stop working out when you need to.

Of course, each woman's pregnancy is unique. Your experiences will differ from mine, as each of my pregnancies was so different from the other, and from those of the other pregnant athletes you'll meet here. Also, your goals will be uniquely personal, as will your fitness level, training goals, your sport, and even where the pregnancy falls in your athletic or competition calendar. But whether you are a recreational athlete, a performer, or a competitor, you can apply the lessons we learned as athletic women and moms-to-be, all the while listening to your body and making the adjustments needed to ensure a fit, healthy, and safe pregnancy. You and the baby will be happier and healthier for your living your life as you know it as long as you can. My only hesitation in sharing my experience and these workouts is that some of you might one day be racing against me! If you pass me while you are pregnant, I will cheer you on and tell you how amazing you are!

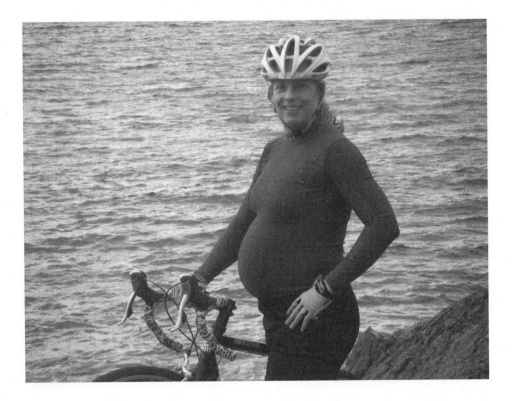

How to Use This Book

If you are like me, you probably just want to flip through and find the sections that seem most interesting or cut to the chase and start the workouts, but it's a good idea to spend a few minutes here learning how to get the most out of *The Pregnant Athlete*. This book is designed for all women who want to stay as fit as they can during pregnancy—the amateur fitness buff as well as the serious competitor. You may already have a training regimen in place for a particular sport or just to stay fit, healthy, and "sexy" (yes, as pregnant athletes we are very sexy). The workouts in this book may give you the confidence you need to keep doing what you are doing or supplement your current program, or you may decide to work out at home more if you don't have a supportive environment at the gym. You can start using this book at any time, whether you are ready to get pregnant or not. In fact, starting early will let you become used to the workouts, become comfortable with identifying your perceived exertion, and establish your own baseline before your body changes.

Most women find it takes about a year to complete the process from conception to getting back on track, and the workouts in *The Pregnant Athlete* provide full-body conditioning throughout the period from preconception to postdelivery. Pregnancy makes quite a few changes in your body—many of them are probably not what you'd expect—and will definitely affect any exercise program you have planned. In addition to providing athlete-focused information about pregnancy and stories about a range of athletes who trained through their pregnancies, this book is designed to help you have a safe, healthy, and active pregnancy. The first step is to know your starting point.

FIRST STEPS

Even if you already know you're pregnant, don't skip the first chapter, "Before You

Conceive." Among other things, it explains how you can gauge your exertion level during pregnancy (your heart rate won't be reliable for that over the next nine months!). It will help you start your athletic pregnancy on the right foot.

Next, share this book with your partner. Some women have partners who are totally fine with their fitness programs during pregnancy. I really lucked out with Steve (although even he admitted to a few moments of concern), and he was a great resource throughout both pregnancies. Others are—perhaps understandably—a little more cautious when they watch the next generation going out for a run before it's even born! Your partner probably already understands how important your fitness is to you, but it will help if he or she understands how working out will actually help you and the baby stay happy and healthy for the next nine months. The book includes some great tips that will help your partner support you and your efforts.

Show the book to your medical team. Discussing your activity level honestly will help them help you. You can bring a sample workout, number of days and amount of time you work out, and your level of intensity. Your physician or midwife can work with you, taking your medical history and current medications (if any) into account, to keep you and the baby healthy. The more information you share, the easier it will be for everyone to be on the same page.

Finally, show this book to your trainer or coach; not all trainers understand the abilities of pregnant women and the exercise modifications you should make as your pregnancy progresses. Remember, maintaining an athletic lifestyle through pregnancy is new to our culture. Even professionals in the training field can be made anxious by the sight of a pregnant woman working out. Help your trainer help you by alerting him or her to your needs.

GETTING STARTED

Each chapter opens with a snapshot of what is going on as your body changes through the months of pregnancy and after delivery. At a glance, this chart shows what to expect, month by month, from seven key points of view:

- Strength: Some women actually get stronger during pregnancy because of hormonal changes and the extra 30 pounds they carry around all day, but your ligaments' ability to support your activities can be compromised.
- Agility: You will definitely see changes here, and not only from the baby bump.
- Stamina: Your stamina and endurance will be affected by many factors during pregnancy.
- Well-being: Hormones play a big part is how you are feeling about yourself and your energy level, both of which play a big role in your workouts.
- Nutrition: Your nutritional needs change over the course of the pregnancy.
- Modifications: As the months go by, you will adapt some of the exercises

and movements to accommodate your changing body shape and abilities.

- Baby's growth: It's good to keep track of how fast your baby is growing.

> "My partner was totally on board. She had gone through it herself a couple of years ago with the birth of our first child, and she trained through that pregnancy. She's also an athlete, a runner, and very fit. She helped me get my workouts in. That made it easier."
>
> —CAROL,
> RUNNER AND MOTHER OF TWO

From there, we'll talk in more detail about workouts, nutrition, and what you can expect each month. I'll share the modifications that allowed me to continue to kick ass in and out of the gym as I progressed through my pregnancies. I can't emphasize enough how much every pregnancy is different from all others! Whether this is your first pregnancy or your fifth, it will be unique. You will have to decide when to make the modifications we suggest along the way. As an athlete, you are used to listening to your body. That goes double for pregnant athletes!

ABOUT *THE PREGNANT ATHLETE* WORKOUTS

Each month I explain how and why pregnancy may affect your body's ability to do the things you are used to doing, and review the modifications most pregnant women should make at this stage of pregnancy. I also share a workout I completed during that period of my own pregnancy. You can "follow along" with my program if you want—all the exercises are explained in the "Exercises" section—but you may find it more useful and fun to build your own workouts with the suggestions we have provided to meet your needs and abilities. The exercise choices, along with the notes on sport-specific modifications, will guide you in working out through your pregnancy.

If you have been training for a while, you will find the structure of these workouts familiar. Even if your trainer has never explained it in these terms, most workouts are likely built on similar principles. The exercises in this book are classified by their function: Squat, Push, Pull, Bend/Hip Flexion, Lunge, Compound Movements, Metabolic/ Conditioning, and Run/Plyometrics. You will also see components of the workouts identified as warm-up, core, and cooldown/ stretch. Each month has suggested workouts; you'll find all of the exercises listed at the end of the book on pages 161–248. Here's how you can put them together to create a plan.

DEVELOPING A WORKOUT PLAN

1. Plan your week.

Establish a rhythm that you can maintain. Pick a start day, depending on your own work and family obligations, and set up your calendar. Do *not* neglect or skimp on your off days!! Creating an activity-rest cycle is more important than ever when you are pregnant. Feel free to make your days off flexible—there may be days when you just don't feel like a heavy workout. Treat that day as an off day and pick up a workout later in the week. Or make it an easier day—it doesn't have to be all or nothing.

Here are a few examples of how you can structure your weeks based on your goals and interests. You can use the same weekly format again and again or vary the formats as you see what fits your schedule and how your body manages the workout load. Based on your schedule and goals, choose the program that fits your needs and abilities.

2. Build your own workouts.

Refer to the "Exercises" section (page 161) and select activities for each strength work-

---

The following examples are based on working out six days a week. Of course you can plan your week around any off day that suits your schedule.

Sample strength training and cardio focus weekly workout schedule. This is a general workout protocol that will benefit any athlete or individual looking to improve her overall fitness who is able to commit to six workout days a week.

Sunday	Monday	Tuesday	Wednesday	Thursday	Friday	Saturday
Off	Strength workout	Cardio	Strength workout	Cardio	Strength workout	Strength and cardio

Sample triathlete focus workout schedule.

Sunday	Monday	Tuesday	Wednesday	Thursday	Friday	Saturday
Off or easy swim	Strength workout and bike	Run and swim	Strength workout and bike	Run and swim	Strength and run	Swim, bike, and/or run (a brick workout)

Sample single endurance sport focus workout schedule. For example, this would be an ideal weekly program for a distance runner.

Sunday	Monday	Tuesday	Wednesday	Thursday	Friday	Saturday
Off	Strength workout and moderate pace sport workout	Speed/ intense endurance sport workout	Strength workout	Moderate distance/ moderate intensity workout	Strength workout— light on the weights	Long, easy distance

out. Each exercise includes step-by-step instructions (illustrated with photographs of our client Jenna, six months pregnant, and me, two years postpregnancy). Based on your time, ability, and level of energy, develop every strength workout to include exercises from at least five of the exercise categories (Squat, Push, Pull, Bend/Hip Flexion, Lunge, Compound Movements and Run/Plyometrics), a metabolic and/or conditioning component, as well as warm-up, core, and a cooldown/stretch. A 30-minute workout might include:

- Two to three sets of one to three Push exercises; include at least one Compound Movement
- Two to three sets of one to three Pull exercises
- Two to three sets of one to three Bend/Hip Flexion exercises

The following examples are based on working out three to four days a week.

Sample strength training and cardio focus weekly workout schedule. This is a general workout protocol that will benefit any athlete or individual looking to maintain or improve her overall fitness. This program is best suited for those who have less time or days to get their workout completed.

Sunday	Monday	Tuesday	Wednesday	Thursday	Friday	Saturday
Off	Strength and cardio/metabolic workout	Off	Strength and cardio/metabolic workout	Off	Strength and cardio/metabolic workout	Off or strength and long easy cardio

Sample triathlete focus workout schedule.

Sunday	Monday	Tuesday	Wednesday	Thursday	Friday	Saturday
Off	Strength and bike workout	Off	Strength and run workout	Off	Strength and run/swim or bike workout	Swim, bike, and/or run (a brick workout)

Sample single endurance sport focus workout schedule.

Sunday	Monday	Tuesday	Wednesday	Thursday	Friday	Saturday
Off or shakeout (easy) cardio	Speed/intense endurance sport workout	Off	Strength workout	Speed/intense endurance sport workout	Off	Strength workout and hard pace sport workout

- Two to three sets of one to three Core exercises
- Two to three sets of one to three Metabolic or Conditioning exercises.
- Cardio component as time permits

You will probably come up with some favorites, but remember that it's important to vary your activities. The ones you like the least are usually the ones that will make the biggest difference in your results. You'll also notice that some exercises appeal to you less at different times in your pregnancy—for instance, you probably won't want to do a Superman (page 200) after the third month! We'll make recommendations for modifications each month—and we also note which exercises are especially helpful for pregnancy health (such as those that strengthen your back and core). You can always switch up your choices according to how your body feels. Just keep in mind: it takes a lot of mental toughness to continue on your training schedule as you become more uncomfortable the "more pregnant" you become.

3. Plan your endurance days.

Every athlete is on a specific schedule based on her sport distance. I had finished up my season racing the Ironman half-distance triathlons so I was accustomed to longer-distance running, swimming, and cycling. As a pregnant triathlete, I focused on the sprint-distance triathlon and strength training. Base your endurance cardio days on your goals for pregnancy and postpregnancy. The sprint distance let me avoid spending too many hours out on the bike or pounding the pavement on runs. I like to keep my baseline volume at 60 minutes of running, 60 minutes of swimming, and 20 to 30 miles of biking. This was easy to achieve and squeeze in, so I didn't feel like I was going to lose everything I worked so hard for over the past ten years of endurance racing. I kept my long slow distance workouts on the weekends so Steve and I could do them together. If you are planning a marathon or longer-distance triathlon after your pregnancy, then you will want to keep your volume up as long as you can during your pregnancy and hope that your body and the baby cooperate. If they do not, don't feel bad about yourself doing the shorter distance or even no distance if you have complications. Your goal for this endurance event is to have a healthy baby and a healthy you for the long run. If you have to modify in ways you didn't expect, keep your eyes on the main goal and keep in mind that you will be back.

4. Prepare your environment.

You can complete the exercises in your gym or living room. But if the weather is fine and you have access to a safe area, such as a public park, take your workout outside. I strongly recommend working out outside when weather and conditions permit, at least for the warm-up and any conditioning routines. I love the fresh air and don't even mind a little rain or, here in New England, light snow. But be careful: give strong consideration to staying inside if it's very hot, humid, or icy.

> "Every book I picked up said to go for a brisk walk. I don't want to do a brisk walk. I've never been a brisk walker. No! So, my approach was to keep doing what I was doing for as long as I could do it."
>
> —GWEN, TRIATHLETE AND MOTHER OF ONE

WORKING OUT

Take a moment to review each workout before you begin. Assemble the necessary equipment and familiarize yourself with the exercises by looking at the pictures and descriptions. A full workout includes these five elements:

- Dynamic Warm-up (see page 15). You should always warm up before exercising, but be especially attentive to this critical first step when you're pregnant. The loosened ligaments of pregnancy make women more susceptible to muscle tears and other aches and pains; warming up reduces the likelihood of injury. There are a wide variety of ways to warm up; we have provided two standard dynamic warm-ups that you can easily memorize and make part of your everyday routine.
- Metabolic/Conditioning. Each workout should include metabolic and conditioning activities to keep the heart rate up and build endurance, balance, and strength. Intersperse two or three sets between, during, and/or after strength sets. Designed to get your heart pumping, they may consist of jogging, jumping, sprinting, crawling, skipping back and forth over a set distance, or performing a set of strenuous exercises (such as Burpees) in place. If you are inside, you may also choose to use a treadmill, stationary bicycle, stairs, or other cardio equipment for the conditioning portion of any workout. Conditioning exercises should be done at a pace that you can maintain during the exercise (an RPE of 6–7); a metabolic exercise should be done at a higher intensity (an RPE of 8–10). (Don't know how to gauge your RPE? See "Before You Conceive," pages 28–29.)
- Strength. The workouts in *The Pregnant Athlete* are designed to be completed in circuit fashion. Go through each circuit as fast as you can with good form, listening to your body and in tune with your level of ability. Work hard, but know your limits. Choose weight loads that allow you to complete the suggested reps but make the last few reps challenging. Strength circuits consist of two or three sets, with the number of repetitions for each exercise given for each set. Select activities from the "Exercises" section (page 161), which provides step-by-step descriptions and photos for each activity, and note the equipment you'll need so you can assemble it before you start (there's a complete equipment list on pages 20–23).

- Core drills. Now is not the time to neglect your core! The exercises we recommend to help you maintain core strength reflect the needs and abilities of your changing body.
- Stretching (pages 18–19). Spend a good 5 to 10 minutes stretching out and/or using a foam roller. It's so good for your muscles, and it feels great!

Look at any of the workouts in the book for examples of how to "build" a workout using this system.

Dynamic Warm-up

Follow one of these two dynamic warm-up routines—or a similar routine you already use—before every workout. Both these routines can be completed inside or outside. Option 1 is ideal for the outdoors and Option 2 can easily be done inside.

Warm-up Routine Option 1 (5–10 minutes)

Equipment needed:

Outside: None. If you have access to a flat outdoor field, court, or sidewalk where you can run and walk back and forth for about 50 feet without obstacles or hazards, by all means go outside. Perform each exercise for one length of your selected distance then jog back to the start point.

Inside: step stool, box, or stairs. If the weather is bad or you prefer to exercise at home, exercise in place. Warm up with step-ups, using a stool or bench, and follow the following suggested times.

ROUTINE

If **outside**, jog your selected distance two to four times.

If **inside**, step up on the box for 1 minute. Alternating feet, step up on box (or to the first or second step on your stairs) with one foot and touch with the other.

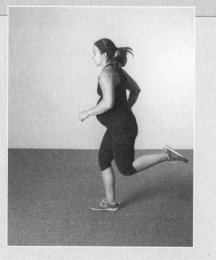

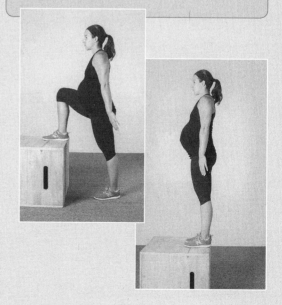

Dynamic Warm-up

Walking Knee Pulls for 15 seconds or your selected distance. If outside, jog to return to start point. If inside, step up for 10 seconds.

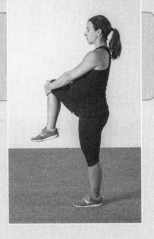

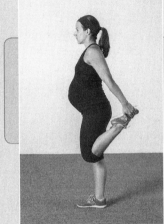

Walking Quad Stretch for 30 seconds or your selected distance. If outside, jog to return to start point. If inside, step up for 10 seconds.

Walking "Chicken Stretch" (piriformis muscle) for 15 seconds or your selected distance. If outside, jog to return to start point. If inside, step up for 10 seconds.

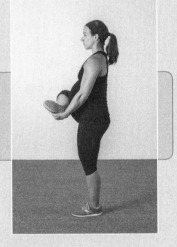

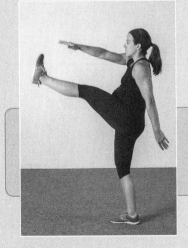

Soldier Kicks for 15 seconds or your selected distance. If outside, jog to return to start point. If inside, step up for 10 seconds.

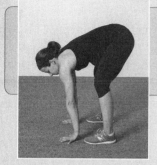

5 to 10 Forward Inchworms: Stand with feet together. Bend down and "walk" your hands out until you are in a push-up position. Drop to a push-up. Walk your feet in to your hands. Repeat.

START

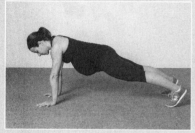
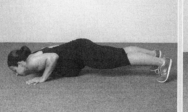
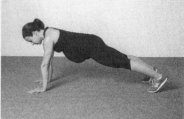

5 to 10 Reverse Inchworms: Stand with feet together. Bend down and put hands on ground. Step feet back; drop to a push-up. Walk hands back to feet. Repeat.

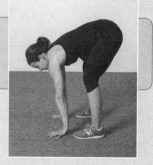

FINISH

Step up for 30 to 60 seconds or jog your selected distance two to four times.

Warm-up Routine Option 2 (5 minutes)

This quick and easy warm-up is ideal for a cardio-focused workout.

   Equipment needed: None.

ROUTINE

Complete 5 rounds of 10 push-ups and 10 squats.

Stretch or Foam Roller Routine

After every workout or exercise session, go through the body stretching the major muscle groups and/or using the foam roller to roll out the major muscles. You can use a foam roller before you warm up as well. Take your time with each stretch and be sure to stretch after every workout while your muscles are warm. Do each stretch first on one side of the body, holding the stretch for 10 to 15 seconds, then move to the second side, holding for 10 to 15 seconds. Then move to the next stretch.

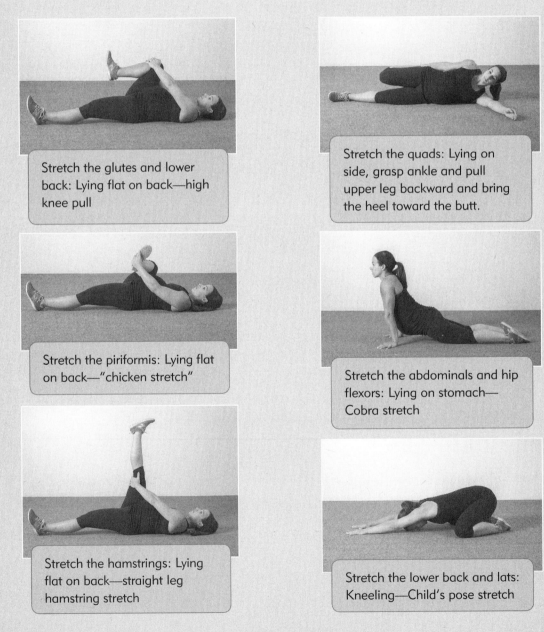

Stretch the glutes and lower back: Lying flat on back—high knee pull

Stretch the quads: Lying on side, grasp ankle and pull upper leg backward and bring the heel toward the butt.

Stretch the piriformis: Lying flat on back—"chicken stretch"

Stretch the abdominals and hip flexors: Lying on stomach—Cobra stretch

Stretch the hamstrings: Lying flat on back—straight leg hamstring stretch

Stretch the lower back and lats: Kneeling—Child's pose stretch

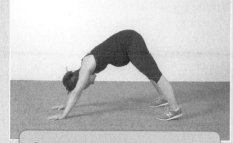

Stretch the hamstrings and calves: Downward Facing Dog

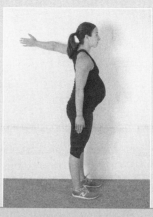

Stretch the chest and shoulder: Standing, use a doorway, wall, or door to push against with an open palm

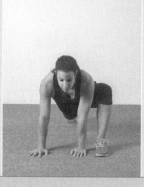

Stretch the hip flexors and groin: Spider-man stretch

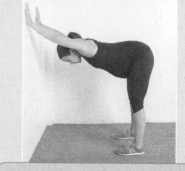

Stretch the upper back: Standing Child's pose

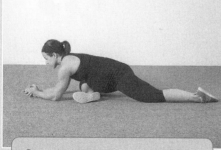

Stretch the piriformis: Modified or regular pigeon stretch

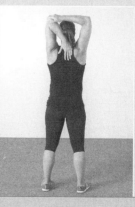

Stretch the triceps: Bend arm over the head and pull down on elbow

Equipment List

The equipment you'll use for the workouts in this book is pretty common—in fact you probably have most of the items around the house already. Adjust your equipment to your workout location. If you are working outside, use resistance bands or tubing in different weights; if you're at home or the gym, take advantage of the dumbbells and kettlebells.

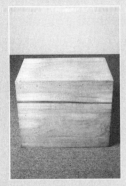

12-, 10-, or 24-inch plyo box. Use a sturdy and stable step, bench, or box. Obviously, lower is easier! You can also use an aerobics step or steps in your house.

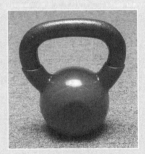

Kettlebells can be used for most exercises calling for dumbbells.

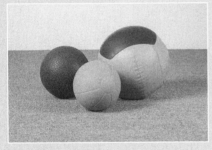

Medicine balls are available in different weights from under 5 pounds to more than 20 pounds. Try different weights for different exercises.

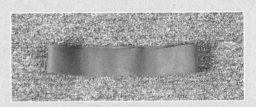

Ankle resistance bands come in light, medium, and heavy resistance. Choose one that is challenging for you.

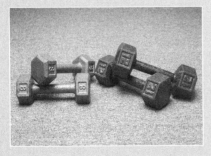

Dumbbells. You will want three sets of dumbbells: light, medium, and heavy, ranging from 5 to 10 pounds to 35 to 50 pounds. A "light" dumbbell is one you can raise overhead for fifteen reps with effort but without straining or losing form. Use "heavy" dumbbells for lower rep sets as well as most lower-body strength moves.

Equipment List

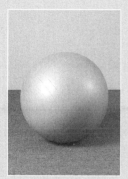

Physioballs are also called Swedish exercise balls. You'll have to pump air into your physioball often to keep the ball tight, so be sure to get a pump that is easy to use.

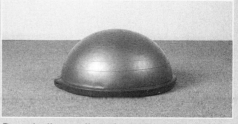

Bosu ball, excellent for balance

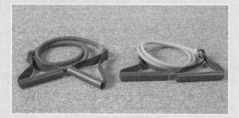

Resistance bands or tubing come in a half-dozen different weights, offering different levels of resistance. You will use at least two different weights—a lighter tube for overhead moves, for example, and a heavier one when you target the larger muscle groups.

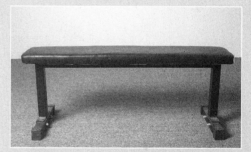

A bench can be used for a variety of exercises, as well as in place of the physioball when stability becomes more of a challenge.

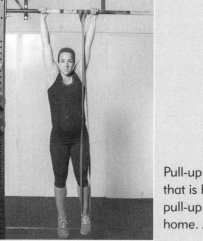

Pull-up bar, a straight bar that can support your weight that is hung from the ceiling, part of a squat rack or pull-up rig, or mounted somewhere in or around your home. A pull-up band can take some of the weight load.

Equipment List

Other equipment you may use either at home or at the gym might include:

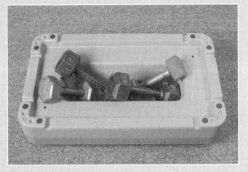

Drive sled. A device or container you can load weight onto or in that can be pushed or pulled

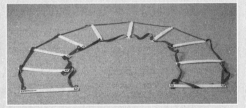

Agility ladder. A flat ladder made of fabric tape. Do not use a household ladder for agility drills!

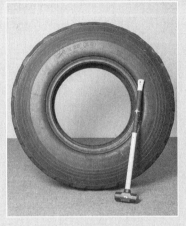

Large truck tire and 8- to 10-pound sledgehammer

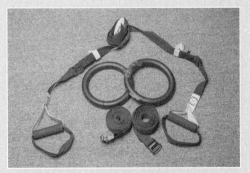

TRX or rings that hang from straps secured on the ceiling

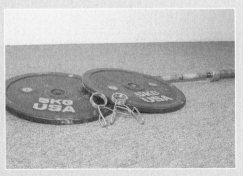

Barbell and weight plates

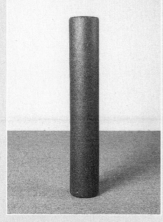

Foam roller, for self-massage of tired muscles

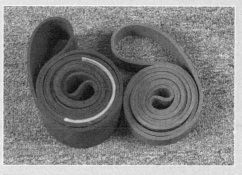

Pull-up bands can be used to decrease the load on your body when doing pull-ups or other body-weight exercises. They can also be used for stretching exercises.

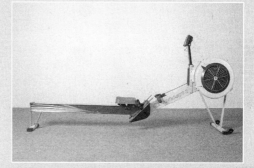

ERG/rower can be used for warm-ups and cardio, as well as metabolic/conditioning sets and exercises. A great non-weight-bearing activity.

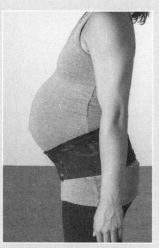

Elastic support belt can help take pressure off the lower back.

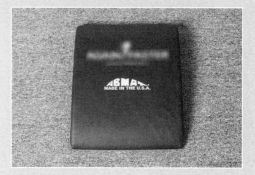

Ab mat can be used to help support the lower back during supine (on your back) abdominal exercises.

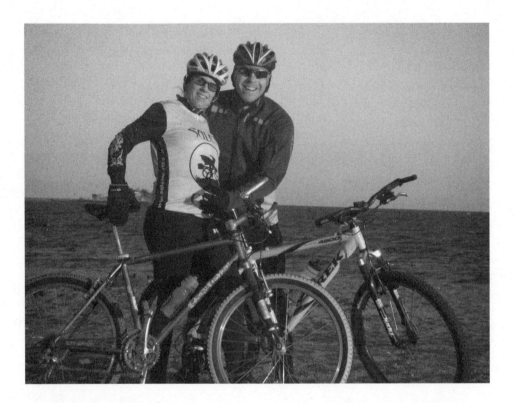

Get Ready for the Event of a Lifetime

Your Body Now

Strength	Continue pushing yourself, and note your current stats in your notebook.
Agility	This is a good time to work on agility and to improve your balance by focusing on single-leg exercises.
Stamina	Get used to using perceived exertion to assess how hard you are working. Note your prepregnancy stats in your workbook.
Well-being	You should feel great!
Nutrition	Establish healthy eating habits now, and learn how many calories you need to maintain your weight at your activity level.
Modifications	Focus on your core and back muscles to strengthen them for the demands of the next year.

In 2007, I was thirty-two years old and had just finished my best season yet in my triathlon career, earning All-American status from USA Triathlon. I had a big decision to make: try to go pro and compete at the next level of triathlon, or step back, stop obsessing over racing, and start a family. I guess I never really quit obsessing over racing, but I did decide to bring more to our lives and "go mom." I stopped birth control one month before the end of this very competitive and focused race year, figuring that if I got pregnant it wouldn't affect my "last big hoorah" season. I'd heard all the old wives' tales, so I figured that once I got pregnant, serious training at my everyday intensity wasn't going to be an option. I didn't plan to focus on hardcore training or racing in the coming months. My plan with that first pregnancy was to keep exercising, but dial it way back on the intensity and get through the first trimester safely. Now that I know better, I can laugh at how people can make you feel guilty for just continuing your regular exercise routine when you're trying to get pregnant. As a rule of thumb, the American College of Obstetricians and Gynecologists considers it safe for women to continue their previous levels of exercise when they are trying to conceive as well as when they are pregnant. Steve was right when he told me, "Giving birth has got to be one of the most intense events you will ever experience. Now is the time to prepare for it, so don't stop working out!" So, if you are considering or planning a pregnancy, get ready now! As an athlete, you know that you perform better at any event when you are prepared and have trained (both mentally and physically). So train for this event by establishing safe and challenging training routines that will maintain or improve your level of fitness now, as you prepare your body for the next year.

CHARTING YOUR BASELINE

If you plan to keep up your current fitness regimen while you are pregnant, take a moment to document what is normal for you now, before you conceive. This might include documenting your swim, bike, and run times at a set distance, your benchmark lifts or workouts—all of which can be easily measured and remeasured before, during, and after pregnancy. If you don't already follow a structured fitness regimen, you might want to start keeping a training notebook.

OLD WIVES' TALE: ATHLETES HAVE A HARDER TIME GETTING PREGNANT.

It's a stereotype that athletic women don't eat enough—in fact, most athletes are pretty in tune with their body and know how important it is to take care of it by eating well. If you do have trouble conceiving, it's likely to have nothing to do with your athletic pursuits—after all, 5 to 10 percent of *all* couples have fertility issues (defined as one year of trying). If you actively attempt pregnancy for six months without success, talk to your physician. If you decide to undergo fertility treatments, many experts advise that you cut back on the intensity and duration of lifting and cardio sessions after IVF treatments.

Write down your prepregnancy age, weight, height, and body fat percentage if you know it. Keep a food diary (or use one of the many free online services) to establish your prepregnancy caloric intake. If you are actively trying to conceive, you can also use this notebook to keep track of your periods and when you have sex. (It may seem memorable at the time, but it's easy to forget later, and these dates will help you determine your due date pretty accurately.)

Now take a look at your routines. The list of activities women should not do while pregnant is actually pretty short, but if your favorite sport is on it then it's a good idea to find something else that will keep you motivated and working hard, especially late in your pregnancy. In this regard I was lucky—as a triathlete I could continue running, swimming, cycling (carefully), and weight training. But even running can be an issue later on for some women, especially if they are short and their belly has nowhere to go but out. The exceptions to the rule of thumb that you can continue doing what you were doing before you got pregnant are mainly sports where you are likely to lose your balance, fall, or suffer impact injuries. If any of these are your go-to sport, start planning alternate fitness routines before you get pregnant:

- Downhill skiing. Pregnant women need more oxygen so they are more likely to get altitude sickness, plus it's harder

CHECKUP WITH DR. HELLER: BEFORE YOU CONCEIVE

If you are a healthy, athletic woman who has decided to have a baby, there's a lot you can do besides simply stopping birth control and starting prenatal vitamins to give your baby the best possible start in life.

As a first step, confirm with your doctor that you are up to date on all your immunizations. A rubella infection during your pregnancy, though highly unlikely, would be very dangerous to your unborn baby. The MMR vaccination protects against measles, mumps, and rubella. It cannot be administered during pregnancy, so it is very important to have the MMR before you conceive. Most physicians advise waiting at least a month after this vaccine before trying to get pregnant.

There has been an increase in pertussis (whooping cough) in children, and vaccination is not possible until after six months of age. Infants must be protected by vaccinating the adults they will be around. TDap is for protection against tetanus, diptheria, and pertussis. The TDap vaccination is recommended for anyone not vaccinated in the past five years who will be with newborns. TDap protects women who are planning pregnancy and will cause them to produce antibodies that can be passed on to their newborn. If you don't get it now, TDap can also be given in the second half of pregnancy; a new protocol has suggested routine vaccination of all pregnant women at twenty-eight weeks.

If you've not been previously vaccinated against hepatitis B, this vaccination would also be ideal before pregnancy, especially for anyone at risk (such as health-care workers).

If you have a medical condition that requires ongoing care, your primary care physician and ob-gyn will work together with you during your pregnancy. For example, women with insulin-dependent diabetes need to manage their condition very carefully before and after they conceive. Insulin requirements will change as the pregnancy progresses and the baby demands more nutrients. It's especially important for women with diabetes who exercise strenuously to monitor their levels carefully and check in with their physicians for testing and adjustments.

to dodge hot dog skiers when your own balance is off.

- Contact sports. Be careful with hockey, soccer, or basketball. "Careful" is the word here after the first trimester. I have a good friend who played soccer until her fifth month and several college basketball players have been in the news for playing until quite late, but most physicians would urge you to find another activity later in pregnancy.
- Scuba diving puts the baby at risk of decompression sickness. Put away your gear for now.
- Horseback riding. A fall or a kick after the first trimester could be very dangerous.
- Trampolining and parachuting expose the mother and baby to injury from falls.

> "My midwife said, 'Keep running for as long as you want to run.' She had a client who ran a marathon and had a baby the very next day. The midwives were really supportive. They said, 'Whatever you've been doing, keep doing it.'"
>
> —GWEN, TRIATHLETE, MOTHER OF ONE

HOW HARD ARE YOU WORKING?

As soon as people learn you're pregnant, you'll start hearing about the dangers of an elevated heart rate and overexertion. Everyone around you will be asking, "Why can't you just start walking? What about yoga?"

Doctors used to recommend that all pregnant women keep their heart rate below 140 beats per minute. They were concerned about maintaining oxygen supply to the baby and keeping body temperature below 102°F. As 140 BPM is actually my training recovery heart rate, this is not a realistic guideline for me if I want a half-decent workout!

As an athlete, you are very familiar with monitoring your exertion level by tracking your heart rate, power, weights, and so forth. You may know your resting, target, and maximum heart rates; your mile repeat paces; or even your Fran time (for those who do CrossFit) like you know your own phone number. You probably have a heart rate monitor—heck, if you're like me you have three or four, with each new version incorporating more stopwatch and GPS features. And you've no doubt heard about that "upper limit" of 140 BPM for pregnant women. So you may be surprised when I tell you that you will need to become just as familiar with a different way to monitor exertion now.

But think about it: Because you're used to monitoring your heart rate, you know that it varies all over the place even when you aren't pregnant, depending on how hot it is, how hydrated you are, and how tired you are both physically and mentally. When you are pregnant, your heart rate becomes an even less reliable indicator of your exertion level. The reason is that the hormones of pregnancy do funny things to a woman's heart rate. Early on, your heart rate after you have begun your exercise bout jumps way up (in fact, a heart rate way out of proportion to how hard you exercise might be the first pregnancy symptom you notice). This situation corrects itself later in pregnancy and then, toward the third trimester, some women's heart rates stay very low no matter how hard they push themselves.

It might be possible to figure out how to compensate for all these changes, but a much better way to monitor your exertion is the Borg Rating of Perceived Exertion (RPE). Developed by Gunnar Borg, PhD, in 1970, this is a subjective rating of how hard you are training, basically a fancy version of the "talk test."

6	No exertion at all (lying down)
7	Extremely light
8	
9	Very light
10	
11	Light
12	
13	Somewhat hard
14	
15	Hard (heavy)
16	
17	Very hard
18	
19	Extremely hard
20	Maximum exertion

Like me, you may wonder why the table starts at 6—why isn't snoozing 0 or 1? The explanation is that if you multiply the numbers by 10, they correlate approximately to the heart rate of a healthy (and nonpregnant) person at different exertion levels. So a rating

"It took me a while to conceive and I did fertility treatments the first time. When I was struggling to get pregnant, everyone said, 'Stop running and gain weight.' And both times, when I actually conceived I was training for a marathon and had just done my 18-mile run!"

—MOLLY,
RUNNER AND MOTHER OF TWO

of 9, representing "very light" exercise, such as walking slowly at your own pace, might correlate to a heart rate of about 90 in "the average healthy person," whoever that is!

We're most interested in the higher end of the scale, of course. A rating of 13 represents "somewhat hard" exercise, a workout that's tough, but it still feels okay to continue. A rating of 17 is "very hard," very strenuous. At an RPE of 17, you can still go on, but you really have to push yourself. A 19 on the scale is an extremely strenuous exercise level. For most people, 19 is the most strenuous exercise they have ever experienced, such as when you are pushing past the finish line in a tough race. If you follow the "times ten" rule, just for comparison, you'll notice that your target heart rate is probably somewhere in that 13 to 15 range, and your maximum is around 18 or 19.

Now that you see the correlation, get familiar with the RPE before pregnancy affects your heart rate. Assess your RPE after your usual workouts and while training at different intensities. Compare your RPE with your heart rate. Get comfortable with trusting yourself to accurately rate how hard you are working so you'll know what to look for as your pregnancy continues.

WHAT SHOULD YOU FOCUS ON?

When you are preparing for a big event you know what to work on—whether it's speed, endurance, strength, or a combination of them all. You know which parts of your body will be put to the test and how much mental power you will need to succeed. Having a baby isn't that different. You have nine months (three trimesters or three mesocycles for those of you who train using periodization) to get ready for the big event—even more if you start preparing your body before you conceive.

Whether it takes you a few weeks or a few months or longer to conceive, put the time to good use. Besides continuing your usual workouts, take advantage of this time to strengthen the areas that pregnancy will strain. Give your lower back, core/midline, and upper body a little extra "love and attention" now—they'll thank you later. And deal with any personal weak spots or imbalances—they will only get weaker when your ligaments relax. For example, during the third trimester when the baby's weight in the front of your body is greatest, the amount of force pulling on your lower back muscles and hamstrings changes dramatically. So use this time and the first two trimesters to strengthen these areas so they are better prepared to manage the additional stress and load. Overall, focus on starting your pregnancy strong, lean, and ready.

"God rigged it wrong—you're most fertile when you are least ready. When I was ready at thirty-five, the fertility gods had different plans for me. It took me a year to get pregnant, with drugs, chemicals, and alternative insemination. I lived in two-week cycles of hope and despair. I wouldn't run for two days, thinking, 'I don't want to jiggle anything out.' A few days later I'd say, 'Dammit, I enjoy these two glasses of wine! I'm not pregnant—I'm going to go out for a 10-mile run.'"

—CAROL, RUNNER, MOTHER OF TWO

SELECT YOUR MEDICAL TEAM

Even though you may not start prenatal visits until the third month of your pregnancy (especially if you have a healthy pregnancy), start shopping around and getting referrals for a doctor or midwife now, before you conceive. Ask your athletic friends with children or talk to women who trained through pregnancy; find out what they liked and didn't like about the medical professionals they worked with. Many doctors discourage high-intensity or serious training during pregnancy in spite of the relaxed guidelines issued by the ACOG in 2002. In fact, many medical professionals who aren't in sports medicine don't "get" serious training at any time, whether you are pregnant or not! Look for doctors who understand your special needs and who will be on your team. Of course, Steve and I wanted a doctor and a practice that would carefully monitor my pregnancy. But we also wanted someone who would actively support my efforts to remain as strong as I could possibly be—ideally someone who was fit and into physical activity, too. So we were very excited when we asked other athletes where they had found support in their efforts to stay active during their pregnancies and several told us about a local practice where most of the doctors are cyclists, runners, skiers, lifters, and adventure enthusiasts themselves. We met and worked with several of their doctors, and found that we had the most in common with and connected with Dr. Joel Heller. It was because of Dr. Heller's advice and support that I asked him to help us write this book.

EATING FOR TWO

If anything, athletes tend to eat healthier diets than most other people do! Still, be sure you

> "I hesitated about getting pregnant. I was nervous—afraid I wouldn't be able to do anything, it's going to be so restrictive, what am I going to do with myself? I know I get kind of nutty if I don't get a good workout in. It's kind of addictive. What was I going to do about that for nine months?"
>
> —GWEN, TRIATHLETE, MOTHER OF ONE

are nutritionally sound and ovulating if you are trying to conceive. Birth control pills and other estrogen and progesterone birth control methods (Depo-Provera, vaginal ring, etc.) may mask any problems with ovulation. Once you go off the pill, if you have regular periods with premenstrual symptoms you are probably ovulating. If you don't have regular periods for three months in a row, work

If you choose to maintain your high level of fitness through your pregnancy, there is really only one person whose buy-in is essential: your partner. That said, plenty of other people will have an opinion about your activities, and they probably will share that opinion with you! There's a huge cultural element to exercise during pregnancy, stemming from different attitudes toward pregnancy itself. The Victorians called it "a delicate condition," and some people still think of it as a disability. Some women complain about the aches and pains of pregnancy and change their tasks at work if they have a physical job. And then there are some cultures where pregnancy is just part of a woman's life, and women keep doing strenuous physical work throughout their pregnancies. So be aware of these cultural differences when you let people know that you are going to continue exercising. Not everyone will understand, no matter how much you try to explain.

Steve

with your doctor to be sure you are meeting your nutrition—especially protein—needs. Because of the requirements of pregnancy, your body must have plenty of protein and fat reserves available for a fetus before it triggers ovulation and allows conception. As an athlete, make sure you consume between 66 and 94 grams of protein a day (depending on your size and activity—about 1.2 to 1.8 grams of protein per kilogram of body weight) and balance your diet with complex carbs and unsaturated fats.

Most doctors and midwives will tell you to start taking prenatal vitamins and omega-3 fish oil three months before you hope to conceive. The folic acid in prenatal supplements helps prevent neural tube defects, which, if they occur, happen very early in pregnancy—that's why it's important to already be taking supplements when you conceive. Prenatal vitamins also provide calcium, iron, vitamin D, and other nutrients that are important for the developing fetus. Your physician may suggest other supplements (such as iron, calcium, and vitamin B_{12}) to accommodate your high activity levels. Don't self-prescribe any supplements—an oversupply of some vitamins (such as A and D) can be harmful to your baby and many supplements have not been tested on pregnant women.

As an athlete, you may already take omega-3 fats to help manage inflammatory

---

TIP: CHOOSING AN OB-GYN

Don't be afraid to shop around! First, ask all your athletic friends who are already moms about their experiences with their doctors. Then when you visit a practice you are considering:

- Be specific about your fitness practices. Rather than saying, "I work out a lot," show your workout log or journal, or explain specifically what your normal routine consists of.
- Ask whether the physicians agree with the ACOG guidelines that support a woman's continuing her normal activities during a normal, healthy pregnancy.
- Confirm that all members of the group practice will support your point of view. You may not be able to see the same doctor every visit.
- Ask whether the doctors follow fitness regimens themselves. Dr. Heller is an athlete. He understands how important my sport is to me. I trusted him to support me in my athletic pursuits while providing guardrails against anything dangerous for the baby or me.
- Share any specific goals (such as upcoming races or events) and your training plans with your medical team.
- Once you have found a medical group with a philosophy aligned with yours, accept them onto your team. Listen when they express caution about specific activities or suggest ways to keep you and the baby safer. Be honest about what you are doing. Follow their advice on hydration, vitamin supplementation, diet, and weight gain.

responses or because you know their role in regulating many physiological functions. It's even more important to take them when you are pregnant. Research has confirmed that adding omega-3 fats to the diets of pregnant women has a positive effect on visual and cognitive development of the baby, and higher consumption of omega-3s may reduce your baby's risk of allergies. Increased intake of omega-3s has also been shown to prevent preterm labor and delivery and lower the risk of preeclampsia and low birth weight.

And keep taking them after you deliver—you'll need them to make breast milk.

Chia and flaxseeds are vegan sources of omega-3s. If you are a vegetarian, vegan, or have other dietary restrictions, your doctor might recommend other supplements, too.

GOOD HABITS TO START NOW

Your body changes fast once you get pregnant. It will be easier to maintain good habits you've already established than to start them if you are feeling a little punky those first few months.

- Eat right. Be sure you eat a variety of healthful foods, and start taking 0.4 milligrams of folic acid and an omega-3 capsule every day. Get used to grazing on complex carbohydrates during the day.
- Notice your RPE during and after every exercise session.
- Drink plenty of water. Stay hydrated; keep your pee the color of watered-down lemonade and avoid "apple juice" color.
- Warm up before and stretch after every workout. When you are pregnant, your ligaments loosen. This can cause joint instability, especially in the lower back and pelvis. Give your body a chance to prepare and recover.

Here's a sample of a typical week's workout schedule before I was pregnant. Because I am a triathlete, my normal week includes "brick" workouts, which are like mini events, including transitioning from one movement pattern to the next. Your week's plans will support your own goals.

Sunday	Monday	Tuesday	Wednesday	Thursday	Friday	Saturday
Off or easy swim	Morning run, strength; evening bike	Morning boot camp run; evening swim	Morning bike, strength; evening short run	Morning track run; evening swim	Morning bike, strength	Morning strength, swim, bike, and/or run (a brick workout)

PRECONCEPTION STRENGTH WORKOUT

This workout offers a challenging routine for the period before you get pregnant. Mix and match this workout with some of the workouts from the next few chapters, for as long as you like until that pregnancy strip changes color, your breasts grow, and you move into the book's overall program. My preconception workout addresses strength, cardiovascular fitness, agility, and balance, while targeting those areas you especially want to strengthen now: your upper and lower back and your core.

Suggested modifications: None. As an athlete you are familiar with what's normal for your own body. Still, pay special attention to your RPE so you can become familiar with using that—not your heart rate—as your gauge of how hard you are working. This workout focuses on establishing your baseline and strengthening your back and core. It will familiarize you with the terminology and routines to come.

In short, while there are no limits to what you can accomplish, here are some good exercise habits you should establish now.

- Drink a glass of water before and after each workout.
- Check in with your RPE.
- Be sure to warm up before each strenuous session, and stretch after.
- Take care of your back by strengthening it and avoiding overstretching.

The Workout

Equipment needed: Physioball; medicine ball; dumbbells; 18-inch step box

Dynamic Warm-up: Check back to the Warm-up (page 15) to refresh your memory.

Conditioning Circuit (2 exercises): Complete this circuit 2 times, moving quickly between exercises

Exercise #1: Medicine Ball Squat Thrust to Vertical Toss (Compound movement)
Reps: 20

Exercise #2: Medicine Ball Chattanooga Push-ups (Core and Push focus)
Reps: 15 per arm

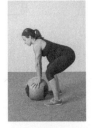

MEDICINE BALL
SQUAT THRUST TO
VERTICAL TOSS

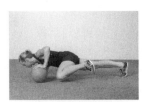

MEDICINE BALL
CHATTANOOGA
PUSH-UPS

Strength Circuit (4 exercises): Complete this circuit 3 times

Exercise #1: Physioball Single-arm, Single Dumbbell Unilateral Chest Press (Push focus)

Reps: 20 per side

Exercise #2: Chest Fly (Push focus)

Reps: 20 per side

Exercise #3: Dumbbell Box Step-up to Reverse Lunge (Lunge focus)

Reps: 15 to 20 per side

Exercise #4: Wood Chops (Compound movement)

Reps: 20

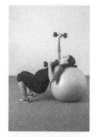
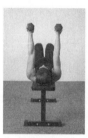
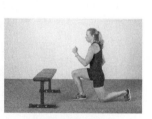
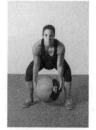

PHYSIOBALL SINGLE-ARM, SINGLE DUMBBELL UNILATERAL CHEST PRESS

CHEST FLY

DUMBBELL BOX STEP-UP TO REVERSE LUNGE

WOOD CHOPS

What's your RPE right now?
Get in the habit of noticing your rate of perceived exertion during and after your workouts.

Core Work (2 exercises): Complete these exercises 3 times

Exercise #1: Physioball Transfer

Reps: 20

Exercise #2: Superman Pulse-ups

Reps: 40

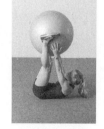
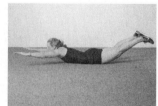

PHYSIOBALL TRANSFER

SUPERMAN PULSE-UPS

Cool Down and Stretch:

Static stretch, mobility work, foam roller: Follow the Stretch Routine on page 18.

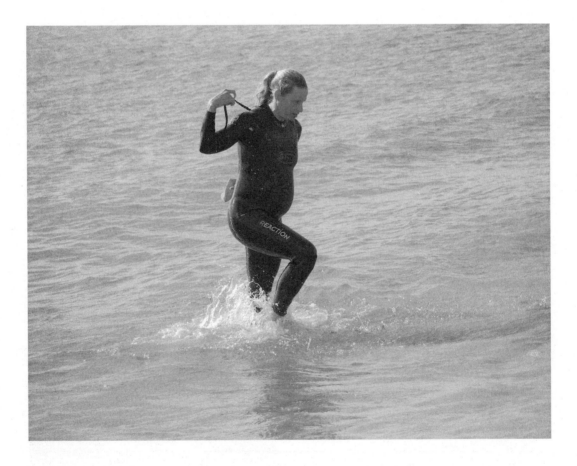

Looking Good, Feeling Great

Your Body Now

Strength	Your ability to lift your body weight or free weights is the same as before your pregnancy.
Agility	Now is a good time to improve your balance.
Stamina	Your heart rate is probably high during and after exercise, so use perceived exertion to gauge how hard you are working. You should be able to work as hard as you did before you were pregnant.
Well-being	Your breasts may be enlarged and tender as you approach the end of Month 1.
Nutrition	Your nutritional needs are unchanged—continue to eat well and establish good grazing and nutritional habits.
Modifications	None. Wear a supportive bra.
Your baby now	At one month, your baby is no bigger than a poppy seed, but the spinal cord, brain, and lungs have already started to develop.

The forty-week pregnancy clock starts ticking with the start of your last period, about two weeks before you conceive. Your first "symptom" of pregnancy might be skipping your period at the end of Month 1. But for some women, the hormonal effects of pregnancy come on so abruptly that they "just know" they're pregnant long before the pee strip changes color. As an athlete, your early tipoff may be an elevated heart rate (compared to what you are used to) during and after exercise, starting about a week after conception. That's your cue to get serious about using RPE to assess how hard you're working.

It's also time to get serious about the "rule of thumb" we've mentioned before: Now that you are pregnant, you can keep doing any activities your body is accustomed to doing. But now is not the time to push to a new level. Don't plan to peak for a race or other competition, and don't even think about making weight for ballet, gymnastics, rowing, or another sport! Just plan to keep training at a healthy plateau from now until you are pushing that baby in the stroller.

OLD WIVES' TALE: WONDERING WHETHER YOU ARE PREGNANT?

Forget about that drugstore pregnancy test kit! Here are some surefire ways to find out whether you are pregnant, courtesy of folklore. Did your dog suddenly start sleeping with you? Do you suddenly not like cucumbers? Are your dreams unusually vivid? Especially dull? Depending on which "old wife" you ask, any of these indicates pregnancy!

SIGNS OF EARLY PREGNANCY

You may sail through your first month without noticing much change, or everything that is going on "under the hood" may show up in the classic signs of early pregnancy. Exhibit A (or B, no make that a C!): Your breasts will almost definitely grow in the first month. Your boobs won't balloon up overnight but they *will* get bigger and they can be very tender in early pregnancy—enough to actually hurt when you run, dance, or do any bouncing movement. As they change size throughout your pregnancy, make sure your bra fits snugly, especially if you're going to exercise strenuously—a well-fitting bra will make you more comfortable now and help prevent sagging later. If your current sports bra doesn't fit well, go buy a larger one—and ask for help getting the right one. If your breasts hurt at night, try sleeping in a light bra or a running bra.

Exhibit P: Your uterus is just a tiny bit bigger than it was last month, but there's not much room for expansion down there and it will start pressing on your bladder very early. That, and your kidneys' improved ability to process fluids, inevitably causes frequent urination and a more "gotta go" feeling. This is *most* annoying when you are running, whether on the track or in field sports. It's that combination of bouncing and being away from "facilities"! Be sure to empty your bladder right before you set out and wear a pad if you need extra protection. I know many women who stopped running entirely because they had to pee after a mile or two every time they ran. I stuck it out for a few months before I decided I had to figure out a way to finish a run without stopping at Dunkin' Donuts to use the restroom. I became very good at finding secluded bushes where I could slide my running shorts over and squeak out those 2 ounces of urine that felt more like 20 ounces. I was pretty proud of myself and Steve was impressed, too. As they say, "Your mileage

CHECKUP WITH DR. HELLER

The earliest you can know for sure that you are pregnant is just before the date of the missed period, about two weeks after conception. This is one reason why it is so important to start the folic acid and fish oil supplementation early. By the time you notice the first symptoms—elevated heart rate when exercising and larger and more tender breasts—you'll already be pregnant.

It's a common—and incorrect—belief that exercise in pregnancy can be harmful. Most first-trimester miscarriages are caused by chromosomal abnormalities, not exertion (although an aggressive fall or impact injury can be dangerous at any time). The notion that exercise might hurt your baby is based on two scientific "faulty connections":

- Doctors used to equate a high heart rate with high body temperature. Overheating is a danger every mother-to-be should avoid, but, as we have seen, heart rates aren't reliable measurements of exertion in pregnancy. Exercise even seems to improve pregnant women's abilities to manage their internal temperatures.
- People are concerned you will fall and hurt yourself and the baby. Later on in your pregnancy, your balance will definitely suffer and you may well fall on your tush, but the chances of hurting the baby in a fall are slim to none.

Early in pregnancy, particularly in the first sixty days, it is very important to avoid hyperthermia—raising your body temperature above 101°F. It is difficult to become so over-heated by exercising that the baby will be harmed, but be attentive to your environment. Don't have an intense or long workout in a warm room, and don't run outside on a hot humid day—early morning and evenings are good times. Stay hydrated and maintain your salt intake. And most doctors advise that pregnant women avoid hot tubs because the high water temperature can cause the body to overheat. So, unfortunately, you will have to forego some of those popular postexercise treats—the sauna, hot tub, or steam room. If you crave a hot soak, take a hot (not scalding) bath instead. More of your body will stay out of the water, and unlike in a hot tub the water will naturally cool down over the course of your bath.

If you like to soak in Epsom salt (magnesium sulfate) baths, consider changing the timing of this treat. Bathing in highly concentrated salt water right after working out (while the pores are still open) has been shown to pull fluids out of the body and cause dehydration. Make sure your Epsom salt soak is at least an hour after you have completed your exercise bout.

So use common sense. Keep cool and hydrated and don't run outside when it's very hot. Avoid sports that expose you to danger or put you in situations you can't control. But there's no need to stop exercising!

may vary!" Pads, convenient Porta-Potties, friendly coffee shops—the important thing is to find a solution that works for you and keep doing your runs.

THE UNDERFILL PHENOMENON

If you fatigue more easily and generally feel tired or lightheaded in the first weeks, it's not because the actual growth processes of pregnancy (growing the baby and the placenta) are so taxing. One of the ways your body is preparing for the baby can make you feel tired, even when you don't think you've worked particularly hard. The condition is called *underfill*—the full term, *vascular underfill*, explains it: your vascular or circulatory system is not filled to capacity. This is the reason your heart rate during and after exercise shoots up so high in early pregnancy. The embryo produces the hormone hCG (human chorionic gonadotropin), which causes your round muscles (namely your blood vessels and digestive tract) to relax. Your blood vessels dilate so your arteries and veins are actually bigger. Your cardiovascular system suddenly has lots more room, but it doesn't have more blood to fill it yet. The system is less efficient and has to pump faster to get the same amount of oxygen where it needs to go.

Other symptoms of underfill are weakness, paleness, sweating, and dizziness. (That sounds like what I encounter during every workout, so these symptoms blended right in with everyday life for me!) Dizziness is a classic symptom of early pregnancy. The sit-

TIP: THE SMELLS OF SWIMMING

If you are a swimmer, you might find the smell of the pool even more off-putting than usual. If you have access to a chemical-free pool, by all means use it, but there is no conclusive research showing that chlorine has harmful side effects on pregnancy. Still, if for no other reason than you will be especially sensitive to smells during pregnancy, you'll want to shower and wash your hair immediately after leaving the pool. Another trick we like to use to help with the taste of chlorine in the pool or of saltwater when swimming in open water is to chew a flavored gum you enjoy. The taste and smell of the gum may mask the other smells. If not, you can put an ointment or menthol rub under your nose so when you breathe in through your nose the smell of the menthol masks the smell of the chlorine.

uation will correct itself by around the end of the fourth month. You'll retain enough fluid to increase your blood volume and you won't feel like you're going to keel over every time you stand up quickly. By the ninth month, your blood volume and cardiac output will have increased by as much as 40 percent! While you're waiting for that, exercise will improve the underfill symptoms by encouraging the growth of red blood cells. It also stimulates the growth of the placenta and the blood vessels supporting it. It's not just a mental thing; it will actually make you feel better.

KEEPING COOL

Because overheating is a big danger for the baby, your body makes several adjustments that help cool you off when you are pregnant. The first sign of pregnancy that many people—like maybe your eagle-eyed grandmother—can actually see is the "rosy glow." Whether you look "radiant" or just feel red in the face, it's a fact that pregnant women have more blood vessels near the skin and they play a big part in dissipating heat. Increased blood volume helps dissipate heat, too, and you might also notice that you will sweat sooner into your workouts.

Exercise also improves your ability to shed excess heat. In fact, pregnancy and exercise work hand in hand to keep you cool. As an athlete, you sweat more than sedentary people and the body temperature at which you will sweat is lowered even more when you become pregnant. And both pregnancy and working out make you breathe harder and take in more air, increasing the cooling effects of gas exchange. And exercise, like pregnancy, increases the amount of blood in your system, which also has a cooling effect.

While exercising improves your body's ability to manage heat, it doesn't give you a pass on avoiding overheating—far from it. A very vigorous workout can increase your risk of overheating, especially if you work out in hot, humid conditions. It is very important to stay cool and well hydrated when you exercise. Drinking plenty of water and paying attention to your environment will minimize the risk of overheating. I was pregnant with Mackenzie in the winter and spring, so I didn't have to worry too much

> "So many people when they get pregnant throw everything they were doing in their prior life out the window and become this new person who doesn't work out and doesn't eat well. If you keep your habits, you feel like, 'Okay, I'm still the same person.'"
>
> —STEPHANIE, SWIMMER, MOTHER OF TWO

TIP: MAKE FRIENDS WITH THE MACHINES

Many people don't like treadmills, the elliptical, or the other cardio machines at the gym—they'd much rather be outside. But late in your pregnancy, you may not feel like running a lot (think pelvic pain, back pain). Or you might not want to ride your bicycle on the road (think balance). So pick a rainy day this month to try out the machines at the gym. Anyone is less efficient when doing a new muscle pattern, and you know how awkward you feel when you first try a new sport or machine at the gym. Trust me, you'll feel ten times more clumsy when you are seven months pregnant! So familiarize yourself with the machines now so you'll be able get a good workout if you need to use them in the last month or so.

about this problem with her. But I carried Maddox through the entire summer, so I always worked out early in the morning or later in the evening and avoided exercise when the sun was at its hottest.

THE FIRST FEW WEEKS

Like many athletic women, during the first weeks of pregnancy I felt strong and had plenty of energy to maintain my normal exercise and life routines. Still, the little voices in the back of your head tend to pipe up as soon as you find out you're pregnant, especially for the first time. It's hard to ignore them when they whisper, "It's time to take a step back." I had just wrapped up my triathlon season at the end of August and was ready for my much-needed off season. I learned that I was pregnant with Mackenzie in September, so the timing could not have been better. With minimal structure, fewer and less intense workouts, Steve and I had figured this was the ideal time for me to become pregnant. My second pregnancy was almost a surprise. No spring chicken (thirty-six years old), I thought it would take me longer to conceive. I had "planned" to conceive in midseason (June or July) but I ended up getting pregnant in March. I wish I had known about Olympic medalist Sonia O'Sullivan, who said, "As for the practicalities while pregnant, I carried on running right up until the day I gave birth. As soon as I found out I was pregnant I just slipped into steady running, 5 to 7 miles a day, which is like walking to most people." You go, girl!

"I biked everywhere up until my due date for all three of my pregnancies. It definitely drew comments from my extended family and from fellow bikers. Some thought I was crazy and let me know they thought I was putting my baby at undue risk. Others cheered me on. My husband certainly knew better than to question my choices."

—ASHLEY, ROWER, MOTHER OF THREE

Before I found out I was pregnant the second time, I had hired a coach to get me through my triathlon season with a bang. I plowed through Month 1 without making any changes to my routines. It was easy: I felt great, and not knowing I was pregnant yet helped! You probably will do the same. Once I found out I was pregnant, I followed through with my coach—I still wanted him to help me prepare for another successful race season, only this time it would be as a pregnant athlete, starting with my first race of the season, the Minuteman Sprint Triathlon in June. When I told my coach the big news, he said, "Congratulations! Okay, I am not going to change your plan. Just do what you can and keep me posted on how you feel."

"Oh boy," I thought, "This is going to be different! But let's do it." Three months seemed like a long way away, and now I had to get there pregnant. I had begun to notice my workouts seemed harder—and indeed they were! What used to be a perceived exertion of about a 13 on the RPE felt like about a 17. My body was changing and so were my

You can continue lifting in pregnancy, but most women benefit from laying off the heaviest weight, especially when doing unilateral strength exercises on the lower extremities. For those not accustomed to low reps and high weight, it's a good idea to maintain your strength with high reps with low weight, and it's not the time to start trying to break through in power lifting! Use common sense. You are already under a certain amount of stress with pregnancy, so don't start doing anything vastly different from what you've done before. Above all, don't start doing a lot of heavy squats. If your pelvic girdle gets overtaxed if can sideline you for months.

Of course, there are always exceptions to the rule. One small study, conducted by Dr. Cooker Perkins and Hannah Dewalt and reported in the September 2011 *CrossFit Journal*, followed two athletes throughout their pregnancies. They each set several strength-related personal records (including Olympic lifts) while pregnant, and both gave birth to healthy babies. I would not recommend all pregnant women shoot for new PRs while pregnant, but you should know that there are women who have seen strength gains during pregnancy without injury.

Some experts caution against high-impact jumping during the early months of pregnancy. As with many pregnancy safety concerns, it is difficult to design a research program that tests the idea without possibly putting women and babies at risk. If nothing else, jumping can stress the abdominal and pelvic ligaments and cause discomfort. You may want to replace box jumps and depth drops (jumping/stepping off an elevated platform) with simple step-ups.

Steve

plans. Suddenly my big season was turning into something quite different!

FIND—AND FOCUS ON—NEW GOALS

One of the biggest changes you will make in early pregnancy is your priorities. No matter what you were focused on before you got pregnant, now you have other goals: a safe pregnancy and a healthy baby. One of the biggest reasons I was committed to continuing to work out was for the health of my baby and myself. Steve and I agreed that stopping what I was doing and "chilling out" for forty weeks would be unhealthy. (In my case it would cause excess weight gain, decreased lean muscle mass, and a bitter and mean personality!)

But even if you don't opt to put your fitness efforts on hold, your priorities certainly will shift, especially if you are a competitive athlete. You are preparing for a completely different "event." It's okay to push yourself, maintain your condition, and even improve your skills and strength. But you shouldn't choose this time to step up your training, reach for new heights, or register for your first Ironman. Be sure you balance exercise with adequate rest. One small way I did this was by finding the closest parking spot to the gym so I could save my energy for my workouts. Take the elevator at work. Get your groceries delivered. You'll find your own ways to take it easy so you can work hard.

Other things may have to give way as you adjust to your new life. "Outsource" some chores to your partner. Skip dinner prep and head for (healthy!) take-out a little more often. I for one took full advantage of my "delicate condition" to grab naps whenever I could during my first pregnancy. Once you have a baby, life will never be the same again. If this is your first pregnancy, enjoy every minute of your peace and quiet!

EATING FOR TWO: START GRAZING

Sure, "eating for two" sounds great! But hold the cannoli! You should plan to gain only a few pounds during the first trimester, and for the first couple of months your caloric intake should be the same as it was before you got pregnant. (I hope you established your baseline to keep yourself honest!) But even though it's not time yet to up your caloric intake from your prepregnancy baseline, it is time to start "grazing"—eating five or six small meals instead of three big meals a day.

Nutritionists commonly advise people who are very active to eat in this way. When you are pregnant, grazing becomes an important strategy to make sure you and the baby get the nutrients you both need, and this goes double if you are working out, for two main reasons:

- When you are pregnant, your liver works to direct sugar to fat storage, so your blood sugar can fall quickly, especially after endurance training.
- If you are nauseous, it is much easier to keep food down if you avoid having an empty stomach and eat more small meals, especially complex carbs.

So, get used to grazing on complex carbs—whole grains, fruits, vegetables, and beans—now, while you have an appetite. Stock your shelves and fridge with these healthy snacks now and purge the house of most of the empty-calorie foods (processed foods in particular). They provide no true nutritional benefit, are high in calories, and often leave you wanting more due to their low nutrient density. Eat at least every three to four hours and have a snack ready to eat during or after exercise. Avoid exercising within 30 minutes of a big meal.

Another important healthy habit isn't about what you eat. Get plenty of rest. You probably already pay attention to your rest–activity ratio to avoid overtraining, but once you are pregnant it assumes a new level of importance. Try to match each hour of exercise with an hour of relaxation.

KERRI WALSH JENNINGS, OLYMPIC VOLLEYBALL GOLD MEDALIST

Kerri Walsh Jennings was five weeks pregnant when she was leaping around in a bikini during the 2012 London Olympics. In a later *Today Show* interview, she explained that she started trying for another baby about a month before the Games. Before she knew it, she had missed a period and was, as she put it, "unreasonably moody." "At some point, you're late and then you start feeling something, and I definitely started feeling something in London," she said.

Dr. Nancy Snyderman, NBC's chief medical editor, says competing at the Games did not increase Walsh Jennings's risk of pregnancy complications. "The risk that she put to herself and fetus was zero to none." Five weeks into a pregnancy, fetuses are tiny, well protected, and "very, very, very hearty," Snyderman says. "The embryo is microscopic. It's just implanted in the lining of the uterus," Snyderman says. "It would take an act of God to dislodge it, not a bump on the tummy, not a dive."

GOTTA LOVE THOSE HORMONES!

Estrogen, progesterone, relaxin, hCG—you'll be reading a lot about pregnancy hormones in the pages of this book. They call the shots for the next nine months, triggering all the changes that prepare your body and nurture the baby. Your hormones will leave no bodily system or organ untouched—your stomach, your blood, your moods, your eyes, even your hair. They will affect your workouts in many ways, some you'd expect and some that will surprise you. Exercise actually enhances some of the adaptations your body makes to ensure your baby's health, such as improving your ability to dissipate heat. But sometimes those pesky hormones will just make your workouts more challenging—for instance, making you feel out of breath especially in the third trimester. Basically you can blame your hormones for almost any-

thing for the next nine months. Resolve now to just think of it as making you stronger. If you can exercise through this, you can exercise through anything!

Even with your hormones raging, the changes of very early pregnancy don't need to affect your workouts much. You may suspect, but you can't know for sure you're pregnant until the end of Month 1. In terms of working out, you can work around most of the changes in your body, and you will treat this month just as you treated your preconception time.

FOCUS ON YOUR CORE

Working on your core in the early months will really benefit you in the long run. Core strength is important during pregnancy, because women can definitely get injured as their bodies change. Hormones (especially relaxin) make pregnant women more prone to dislodged or dislocated joints if they haven't been working on strength. Focus on the core: the abdominals (rectus, oblique, and transverse), the back (erector spinae) as well as your butt (gluteus maximus). Women who have had good strength training before getting pregnant are less likely to get injured, but no matter how strong you are, it's still important to avoid stressing the pelvic ligaments by overlifting.

> "My regular routine before and after pregnancy was dancing/teaching three times a week, four to six hours a day, plus yoga, plus rehearsals. When I got pregnant, I pretty much stopped rehearsing but continued teaching. I stopped dancing in Month 9."
>
> —MEGHAN, DANCER, MOTHER OF ONE

HOW MUCH SHOULD YOU WORK OUT?

By the time I got pregnant the second time, I had learned much of the message of this book and I knew I could continue to work out at an intense level, even though I did opt for a reduced schedule. Of course, as a fitness professional, my "reduced schedule" of one to three hours each day, five to six days a week may seem like a lot to most people! Few women have the time or desire to work out three hours a day, even if they're not pregnant! Your routine will suit you and your sport or activity. So figure out what works best for you and try to stick with your normal schedule as much a possible.

Most women find an hour-long workout to be optimum, and the workouts in the book are designed to take about that long.

The modifications in this month's workouts focus on timing your workouts for the periods of your day when you feel best. For instance, if you tend to feel ill in the morning, then move your workout to later in the day when you have eaten and feel stronger.

One important note for now and throughout your pregnancy: Keep hydrating. Don't be tempted to drink less because it makes you have to go to the bathroom. Drink until your urine runs pale yellow or clear.

Here's what a typical workout week looked like for me in the first month. Basically, it is the same as before conception.

Sunday	Monday	Tuesday	Wednesday	Thursday	Friday	Saturday
Off or easy swim	Morning run, strength; evening bike	Morning boot camp run; evening swim	Morning bike, strength; evening short run	Morning track run; evening swim	Morning bike, strength,	Morning strength, swim, bike, and/or run (a brick workout)

MY MONTH 1 STRENGTH WORKOUT

Suggested modifications: Modify by finding the best time of day to work out if you have morning sickness (or nausea at any time of day). Most women don't have bad morning sickness in Month 1, but if you do feel nauseous you won't want to do any exercises with your head below your belly—skip the pike presses and do shoulder presses instead. Your blood oxygen level is low—if you train at unaccustomed high altitudes you might get an early tip-off that you're pregnant! If you are like most women, you won't even know you are pregnant at this early stage, so no modifications are necessary either in exercises or in sports. Balance and ligament stability are not affected yet, so biking, running, and trail running are fine. If you are a swimmer, you can look forward to enjoying this activity right up to delivery. If any activity makes you uneasy, reassess your goals and consider an alternative, but if you feel great, as I did, keep at it!

Single-leg exercises in these early months will help you improve your balance. Later on you'll be glad you did this.

The Workout

Equipment needed: Agility ladder; physioball; barbell, dumbbells; medicine ball

Dynamic Warm-up: If you need to refresh your memory, check back to the Warm-up on page 15.

Conditioning Circuit: Complete this circuit one time, moving from one exercise to the next, resting only as much as you need to.

Dot Hops

Double-legged plyo-hops forward and backward
Double-legged plyo-hops lateral (side to side)
Single-leg (leg 1) plyo-hops forward and backward
Single-leg (leg 2) plyo-hops forward and backward
Single-leg (leg 1) plyo-hops lateral (side to side)
Single-leg (leg 2) plyo-hops lateral (side to side)

Reps: 30 seconds each

DOT HOPS

Strength Circuit (7 exercises): Complete this circuit 3 times

Exercise #1: Barbell Split Squats (Squat focus)
Reps: 10 per leg

BARBELL SPLIT SQUATS

Exercise #2: Yogi Push-up (Push and Core focus)

Reps: 10

Exercise #3: No-Touch Step-ups (Squat focus)

Reps: 20 per side

Exercise #4: Box jumps (Plyometric)

Reps: 15

Exercise #5: Medicine Ball Straight-legged Ab Pulses (Core focus)

Reps: 50

Exercise #6: Physioball Single-arm DB Row (Pull focus)

Reps: 15 per side

Exercise #7: Plank Single-arm Dumbbell Reverse Fly (Pull focus)

Reps: 15 per side

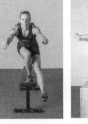 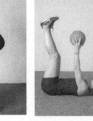 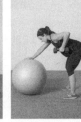 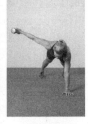

YOGI PUSH-UP | NO-TOUCH STEP-UPS | BOX JUMPS | MEDICINE BALL STRAIGHT-LEGGED AB PULSES | PHYSIOBALL SINGLE-ARM DB ROW | PLANK SINGLE-ARM DUMBBELL REVERSE FLY

Metabolic Circuit: 10-9-8s of Medicine Ball Slams with Sprints

Reps (Complete with as little rest as possible):
10 slams, then sprint out 30 to 40 yards > walk back to ball
9 slams, then sprint out 30 to 40 yards > walk back to ball
8 slams, then sprint out 30 to 40 yards > walk back to ball
Repeat the pattern all the way to 1 slam with a sprint.

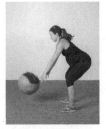

MEDICINE BALL SLAMS

Cool Down and Stretch:
Static stretch, mobility work, foam roller: Follow the Stretch Routine on page 18.

Looking Good,
Sucking Wind

Your Body Now

Strength	Your strength is unchanged, but don't overtax your pelvic muscles.
Agility	You may notice some softening of your joints, and you may be extra flexible.
Stamina	Your heart rate is probably high during and after exercise, so use perceived exertion to gauge how hard you are working. You should be able to work as hard as you did before you were pregnant. Possible fatigue, lightheadedness.
Well-being	Your breasts are probably enlarged and tender. You may have morning sickness. You may experience some mood swings or anxiety.
Nutrition	Your nutritional needs are unchanged—continue to eat well and establish good grazing and nutritional habits. Eat complex carbs to avoid constipation.
Modifications	Time your workouts for when you feel best. Use lighter weight in squats and avoid deep squats if you feel "overflexible."
Your baby now	The baby is about the size of a raspberry, about 0.6 inch from head to butt; major organs including the genitals are forming.

Wow! You just found out you're pregnant, and you're already starting Month 2! Trust me, the time won't fly by so fast toward the end of your pregnancy, so enjoy it now. The baby is still very small—about the size of a blackberry—but some of the things happening in your body are extremely noticeable, at least to you! Your breasts are still expanding, and probably pretty tender and sensitive. You often feel tired and you might want to sleep more. You know the shortest route to every bathroom in your office building (or discreet bush on your regular run).

Other changes are still under the radar but that doesn't mean you don't need to take them into account. Early in pregnancy the hormones progesterone and relaxin work together to soften cartilage and loosen your joints. Your pelvic area is especially vulnerable because it is already preparing for the baby's trip down the birth canal. You may notice some pain or a "just not right" sensation in your pelvic girdle or sacroiliac joint, or your knees after a long run, or you may experience extra soreness after a workout with single-leg squats or lunges. Consider adjusting your routine so any lifting you do can help, not hurt, your program. Go a little lighter in weight and avoid very deep squats (10 degrees or more below parallel) with weights. This adjustment should allow you to continue with these movements until the third trimester or even the end of pregnancy.

Progesterone and relaxin do their job in your gastrointestinal tract too. With the muscles "down there" more relaxed, food moves more slowly through the system. Good for the baby: slower digestion means that more nutrients are absorbed. Bad for you: it means indigestion, heartburn, bloating, and constipation. Be sure to eat plenty of fiber and complex carbohydrates. You may also find that food that never gave you trouble before now causes gastrointestinal distress. Those foods are in your system longer, exposing your body longer to their nutrients and chemicals. This is yet another reason to drink lots of water (just keep your pee on the light-colored side).

OLD WIVES' TALE: IF YOU HAVE NO MORNING SICKNESS, IT'S A BOY. IF YOU ARE SICK ALL THE TIME, IT'S A GIRL.

There are so many old wives' tales predicting your baby's gender, you can pick the one you like best!

You might have a boy if your right breast is larger, you crave meat and cheese, the hair on your legs grows very fast, you are clumsy, your legs get big, or you dream of a girl.

On the other hand, you might have a girl if your left breast is larger, you are more graceful than usual, your legs stay lean, or you dream of a boy.

If your pee is bright yellow, it's a boy; if it's dull yellow, it's a girl. If your pee is dark, you aren't hydrating enough!

THAT QUEASY FEELING

Probably the most famous—or infamous—side effect of early pregnancy is morning sickness. It makes some women so nauseous that they have to nibble soda crackers and sip water before they can even get out of bed in the morning. A quarter of pregnant women never have "morning sickness" at all, but if you are in the unlucky 75 percent, then you know that morning sickness isn't just for the morning! An upset stomach can strike at any time of the day. Some women actually feel so bad that they lose a pound or two during the first trimester, instead of gaining a few pounds as most women do.

CHECKUP WITH DR. HELLER

Morning sickness starts to appear in earnest around four weeks from conception (six weeks from the last period). Its severity ranges from light to debilitating. (Luckily, cases of severe and intractable morning sickness requiring medical intervention [hyperemesis gravidarum] are very rare, but if you lose more than 5 pounds, contact your health provider.)

Of course, "morning sickness" is a misnomer—some of my patients tell me, "I feel horrible all day long!" And I have many athletic patients who, unlike Brandi, just have to lay off for a while. They just don't have the energy—or the ability to eat—to do their usual routine. Face it, you can only do what you can do. Sometimes you just have to sit things out until you can begin to get enough calories to give you energy. Brandi was fortunate, but there are some people who just don't have a choice. It's not a question of mind over matter.

As bad as you may feel now, don't feel like you're never going to get better or you're not going to ever work out again! The good news is that in almost all cases it's going to get better before enough time elapses to erase your fitness gains. If you feel awful, look at the first trimester as a mini-vacation and enjoy not pushing yourself for a few weeks. For now, cut back on the intensity or weights and then pick things up again in the second trimester, when most women have plenty of energy and feel great.

Do continue to do short workouts, even if you feel lousy. There's plenty of evidence that they will help you feel better almost immediately. For other morning sickness remedies, see the box on page 53.

Don't worry if this happens to you—unless you are in the very small number of women who suffer from extreme morning sickness requiring medical intervention, the lack of weight gain now won't jeopardize your baby's health. The weight you gain in the first couple of months represents your fat reserves, not the baby or the placenta. And rest assured that the baby is first in line for any nutrients you take in.

I was very lucky as far as morning sickness was concerned—I felt fine and had a good appetite in the mornings, so I glided through my workouts without any queasiness slowing me down. But in the afternoon and evening, now that was a different story! Before I got pregnant, I loved chicken, pasta, and . . . basically everything. But when I was pregnant with Mackenzie, just the thought of eating grilled chicken or even any of my usual dinner choices made my stomach turn. And if just thinking about a food made me nauseous, I sure didn't want to eat it! I turned into the world's pickiest eater, especially at suppertime. Every night I had to look around for something to eat that wouldn't make me feel sick. The result: many not-so-exciting dinners. I am talking about crackers, sub shop subs (I never liked these before I was pregnant), ice-cream sundaes, or even pancakes. My new food choices even tipped some of my friends off to my pregnancy before I was ready to share the news.

If you are one of the many women who follow a particular method of eating (vegetarianism, the Zone diet, Paleo), recognize that your appetite and desire for certain foods may change dramatically when you are pregnant. The foods you love may become foods you can't tolerate, and you may begin to seek out and crave things you previously had no desire to eat. My new favorites were jelly doughnuts, bismarcks, and cheese steak subs. Don't get discouraged if your goal of eating Paleo, Zone, or Mediterranean goes out the window. Regardless of what foods you seek out, just do your best to focus on the big picture of eating a diet that is as well balanced, colorful, and natural as possible. You can return to your food plan when your hormones are back to normal—about 8 months from now. (Meanwhile, if you have been following a Paleo or higher protein and lower carb diet and you revert to eating an increased percentage of your diet from carbohydrates, you will see a faster increase in body weight. This is water, not fat. When you introduce more carbohydrates in your diet, your body stores more water. For every gram of carbohydrate you take in, your body retains 4 grams of water.)

> "I did a half Ironman a week after I found out I was pregnant (my eighth week). I'd trained all summer so of course I did the race! I did not just train all summer to not do this race! After the race, did I relax? No. I can't. I mean, I've been working out for so long, it's been such an important piece of my life. I couldn't really bear the thought of not doing it."
>
> —GWEN, TRIATHLETE, MOTHER OF ONE

Food aversions don't affect all women, but they can pose extra hurdles when you are trying to fuel your workouts in addition to the baby's growth. Try to eat enough calories to enable you to perform the tasks you need to do: exercise and develop that baby without gaining excessive fat. (Note that I did not say to avoid gaining *weight*; you need to gain *weight* in fluids and appropriate amounts of fat for your health and the baby's.) Luckily, most food issues will be over by the third or fourth month, giving you your appetite back when the baby really needs the extra calories. Meanwhile, eat lots of small meals with complex carbohydrates to regulate your blood sugar and keep something in your stomach.

If you have morning sickness or other early pregnancy side effects, look on the bright side—these are the classic symptoms of a healthy pregnancy. Feeling sick and fatigued is a sign that your hormones are doing their job and all systems are "go"! Don't let these symptoms become excuses for skipping your workout. Most women report that even when they don't want to drag themselves down to the gym, they actually feel better after working out. Do what you can—a light workout or a short run or ride. Just remember that your workouts—strength training, running, swimming, cycling, boot camp, or CrossFit—are a means to an end at this point. The more you can stick with your routine, the better you'll feel, the stronger you'll be, and the sooner, better, and faster you will return after your baby is born.

If working out to keep yourself happier, healthier, and more balanced isn't enough, here's another benefit of first trimester exercise that you can use to motivate yourself when you feel like taking it easy: Exercise in early pregnancy enhances the normal adaptations your body is making. By imposing an extra burden, it increases the growth and improves the function of the placenta. This prepares the placenta for stresses later on, either planned, such as exercise, or unexpected such as an accident or blood loss.

FUELING YOUR WORKOUTS

If you've been athletic for a while, you are probably pretty aware of how much and what kinds of food you need to eat to stay strong. It's even more important to choose your foods carefully now, when you may not feel like eating a wide variety of foods. Even though I was a fairly picky eater in my first pregnancy, I tried to focus on eating enough

TIP: DEALING WITH MORNING SICKNESS

No one knows exactly what causes morning sickness, but here are some tried-and-true ways to feel less miserable during these first few months.

- Sniff a lemon or a sprig of fresh rosemary or mint (put one in your pocket or purse). Nausea is often triggered by smells, and your higher levels of estrogen make your sense of smell more sensitive.
- Drink plenty of water. This may seem counterintuitive, but dehydration increases nausea. Hot or cold drinks are easier to drink than lukewarm ones. Crunch ice cubes or eat Popsicles.
- Eat smart. Salty snacks will settle your stomach and make you thirsty. Keep plenty of bland carbohydrates handy—crackers, dry cereal, pretzels. If liquids are easier to keep down, drink smoothies.
- Graze. Eat a lot of small meals so your stomach doesn't get empty, and don't eat too much at once. Eat before you get hungry.
- Carry a toothbrush and breath mints.
- Get plenty of sleep. Many women report that morning sickness is worse when they are overtired.

of the right things to help me through my day as a mom and as an athlete. For example, I would start each day with my vitamins, snack on healthy nuts and fruits, plan out a well-balanced dinner, and be mindful of any empty-calorie food that I was craving. Sometimes I indulged myself, but most of the time I found a (slightly) healthier substitution.

> "I never had any problems with my ligaments, but I did notice that I was *very* flexible. The bottom of my squat was just crazy—I was sitting on my heels, perfectly comfortable! But I never noticed any weakness or instability in my joints."
>
> —HEATHER, CROSSFITTER, MOTHER OF TWO

Most women pay attention to their calcium intake, but remember that you need extra now. Besides the normal turnover in your own skeletal system, the baby's bones and teeth will be growing too. Be sure to get 1,000 mg per day either from a supplement or dairy products. And get 600 IU of vitamin D by spending time outside or by taking a supplement.

When you are training and pregnant to support your needs and the baby's growth, be sure to get plenty of protein to support your needs and the baby's growth. Ordinary sedentary women need 46 grams of protein a day. Pregnant women, even those who aren't training, need 71 grams a day (most Americans meet this requirement in their normal diets). You need even more—according to Lauren Antonucci, MS, RD, director of Nutrition Energy in New York City, pregnant women who are very active need about 10 more grams of protein than they did before they conceived. Find protein in lean dairy and meats, poultry, fish, beans, and eggs. If you are a vegan and you lose your taste for vegan-friendly high-protein foods, you may need to consider a protein supplement—but be sure to talk with your doctor first. Regardless of the source, as a very active *and* pregnant woman, a good rule of thumb is to consume about 1.8 grams of protein for each kilogram of body weight.

As you go through the first trimester, you may continue to get lightheaded when you stand up too quickly, because your blood volume doesn't fill your newly relaxed circulatory system. Your body needs iron to manufacture all the new red blood cells that will eventually fill that space—twice as much iron as you needed before you got pregnant: 27 milligrams a day. Eat plenty of lean red meat, poultry, and fish, and iron-fortified foods, such as orange juice. If you are following a diet that restricts these items, talk to your physician or medical team about iron supplementation.

Get used to your new eating habits—cutting out alcohol, eating less of the big fish, and taking a multivitamin and some fish oil or other omega-3 supplement daily.

FOODS TO AVOID DURING PREGNANCY

Even as I encourage you to eat more and a wide variety of foods, there are some kinds

> "Within three weeks of finding out I was pregnant, the oxygen level went way down. It was like I had never run in my life. That was all through the first trimester, when I also had terrible morning sickness. I ran through morning sickness—it really does make you feel better. Before you start, you think, 'How can I get out there and move?' But working out, even lightly, definitely helps. When you hit that second trimester, you think 'Oh—my air is back!'"
>
> —MOLLY, RUNNER, MOTHER OF TWO

of foods you should stay away from for the next nine months. The Mayo Clinic suggests you avoid these foods that might adversely affect your health or the baby's:

- Seafood that is high in mercury. Avoid large fish, such as swordfish, shark, king mackerel, and tilefish, and tuna steak. Fish is a great source of omega-3 fatty acids, so do eat 8 to 12 ounces of shrimp, crab, canned light tuna, salmon, pollock, catfish, cod, or tilapia per week.
- Raw or undercooked seafood, including raw oysters and clams, refrigerated lox (shelf-stable lox is okay), and sushi.
- Undercooked meat, poultry, and eggs. You are more at risk for bacterial food poisoning when you are pregnant.
- Unpasteurized foods. Make sure the labels on soft cheeses say "pasteurized."
- Unwashed fruits and vegetables, raw sprouts.

- Large amounts of vitamin A. The recommended amount for pregnant women is 2,565 IU daily. Three ounces of beef liver contains ten times that amount.
- Caffeine. Limit coffee to two cups a day, or tea to four cups a day. Don't drink herbal teas (even those marketed to pregnant women).
- Alcohol. No level of alcohol has been proven safe during pregnancy.

WORKING OUT

During my first pregnancy, I cut back to a much less intensive routine. Still, I had signed up for the Philadelphia half marathon, scheduled at around my Week 12, so I trained lightly and planned to go easy on race day. The second time around, the timing was similar, but my attitude and approach were very different. During pregnancy number two, I wasn't just planning to jog along; I was following a training plan to compete in the Minuteman Sprint Triathlon at the end of my first trimester. I had hired a coach before I knew I was pregnant and I was in full race mode. My coach's plan for each week was pretty intense, including long runs, speed work, open water swims, biking, and "brick" workouts. I gave it my best shot, but I didn't stress about not getting in 100 percent of what he had planned for me. My attitude was: I will be happy with whatever I can get in!

I will admit, it was incredibly frustrating to follow a training plan, all the while knowing I wouldn't get any faster, just slower! But

---

JOAN BENOIT SAMUELSON: GOLD-MEDAL OLYMPIAN MARATHONER

Joan Benoit Samuelson was still in college when she set a women's world record of 2:35:19 in the 1979 Boston Marathon. She won again—and set another record—in 1983, then took a gold medal in the 1984 Los Angeles Olympics.

In 1987, she became one of the first elite athletes to openly compete while pregnant, when she completed the 1987 Boston Marathon at three months pregnant with her first child. She didn't win, but she posted an amazing time! "I see myself as having a responsibility to lead as strong a life as I possibly can," she told *Runner's World.*

---

you know, in the big picture I was totally fine with that and just took it as a personal challenge to see if I could keep going and do what I do. Even though I was only two months pregnant, my routine was already a lot more challenging. What had been an effort of about 14 before I got pregnant now seemed like a 16, and I could only imagine what Month 9 would feel like. I quickly learned it was better to not think about how I would feel in the future, just stay in the moment of every workout and take each one, day by day, month by month, and hope for the best. Like all pregnant athletes, I had to get used to the changed relationship between my heart rate and the RPE scale—all I knew at first was that what used to be easy was now hard.

It's all part of the phenomenon of racing and training through a pregnancy. You have to accept that even though you will get stronger (after all, you will be carrying 25 to 35 more pounds everywhere you go by the end) you won't *feel* stronger or move faster for the next nine months. And face it, even though

you can, with work, maintain your muscle mass, you will gain some fat. These are the realities of a healthy pregnancy. What's key here is the baby's health. You just have to accept the extra pounds and work through it all knowing that by maintaining your activity and fitness you will be able to get back to your prepregnancy shape after you deliver.

This month's workout takes into account the developments underway in your body. Steve often reminded me of the need to "cross-train" for pregnancy. If you are a runner you may need to spend more time doing additional strength training exercises, whether at the gym, outside, or at home. Regardless of your sport, biking, running, swimming, field sport, or other, you will soon learn to appreciate the value of adding in some weight-bearing routines as the weeks go by. Like any other "event," pregnancy works some muscles at the expense of others. Your lower back, chest muscles, and hip flexors will be shortened over the course of the pregnancy because of the weight of the baby carried in front of your body. The same dynamic will stretch the hip extensors, hamstrings, glutes, abdominals, and upper back. Focus on strengthening those stretched muscles. And be sure to take time in your post-workout routine to stretch out the muscles that pregnancy will shorten.

But bear in mind that, if at this point you do not need to modify your exercises, don't. There is no need to modify your activity and workouts if you don't have to. That time will come soon enough. So listen to your body and notice how it reacts to each workout.

This is also the time to really focus on getting adequate rest to ensure your post-workout recovery—it's just as important as eating well!

The Month 2 workout schedule below is pretty similar to the one for Month 1. For me, early pregnancy affected the intensity of my workouts more than the frequency.

Sunday	Monday	Tuesday	Wednesday	Thursday	Friday	Saturday
Off or easy swim	Morning run, strength; evening bike	Morning boot camp run; evening swim	Morning bike, strength; evening short run	Morning track run; evening swim	Morning bike, strength	Morning strength, swim, bike, and/or run (a brick workout)

MY MONTH 2
STRENGTH WORKOUT

Suggested modifications for Month 2: If you are nauseous or lightheaded, time your workouts for the times when you feel at your best. Or cut back or take a day off until you feel better. Be sure you eat enough beforehand so you can maintain your routine, but also to ensure that you're getting enough calories every day. Eat at least as much as you did when you were working out and maintaining your weight before you got pregnant. This can be challenging if your stomach is upset—eat light meals, and see the tips on page 53 for more ideas.

There can be some softening of the joints in early pregnancy, so go easy on the weight for deep squats or lunges.

The baby is still safely tucked below the pelvis and your center of gravity is unchanged. Still, if you are a cyclist, a good practice to start now is bringing your cell phone with you on rides and, if you don't already, wearing a Road ID or similar product that includes your contact info and emergency info as well as your ob-gyn. This may also be a good excuse to get another bike. If you only own a tri-specific bike, you may consider looking to buy a road bike—one that is a bit more stable and puts you in a better position to brake and change gears without having to take your hands off your bars.

The Workout

Equipment needed: Barbell, medicine ball; resistance or tubing band; dumbbells; physioball/ bench; pull-up bar

Dynamic Warm-up. Refer to page 15 if you need to refresh your memory.

Conditioning/Metabolic Circuit: Complete this circuit one time with as little rest as possible
Sprint 50 yards; run backward to start position > 20 Burpees
Sprint 50 yards; run backward to start position > 15 Burpees
Sprint 50 yards; run backward to start position > 10 Burpees

Strength Circuit #1 (1 exercise): Complete the prescribed reps

Exercise #1: Standing Barbell Overhead Press (Push focus)
Reps: 8/6/4/2 with 90 seconds rest between sets

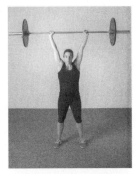

**STANDING BARBELL
OVERHEAD PRESS**

Strength Circuit #2 (2 exercises): Complete this circuit 3 times

Exercise #1: Air Squat to a Pull-up
(Squat and Pull focus)

Reps: 10

Exercise #2: Forward Lunge with
Single-arm Dumbbell Snatch
(Lunge and Compound
Movement focus)

Reps: 12 of each arm and leg

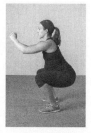

**AIR SQUAT
TO A PULL-UP**

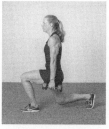

**FORWARD LUNGE
WITH SINGLE-ARM
DUMBBELL SNATCH**

Metabolic Circuit: Mountain Climber Tabata
4 minutes/8 rounds total: 20 seconds work,
10 seconds rest, repeat.

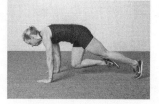

MOUNTAIN CLIMBER

Cool Down and Stretch:
Static stretch, mobility work, foam roller: Follow the Stretch Routine on page 18.

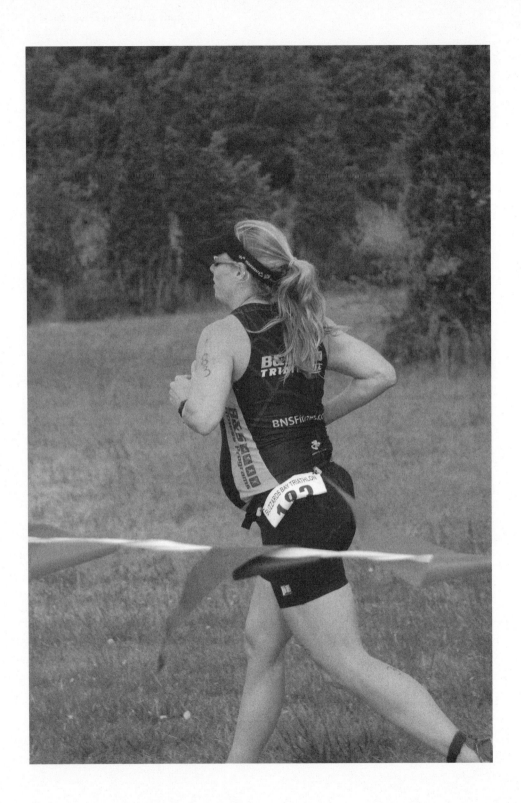

Working Out for Two

Your Body Now

Strength	You are as strong as ever; you can even increase stable joint lifts, such as front and back squats and deadlifts
Agility	Relaxin reaches its peak at fourteen weeks, so be alert for softening joints and ligaments.
Stamina	The baby's position and your hormones can cause shortness of breath.
Well-being	You may be experiencing morning sickness. Your moods may swing between calmness and irritability and you may be forgetful. Your sleep may be disrupted by restless legs and leg cramps.
Nutrition	Eat small meals to fuel your workouts through any morning sickness.
Modifications	Time your workouts for when you feel best in the day. Protect your lower back by putting your hands under your butt for leg lifts.
Your baby now	At three months, the baby is about the size of a lime, a little more than 2 inches from head to butt. Teeth and nails, bones, and muscles are appearing.

For a pregnant woman in her thirties, there is nothing more nerve-racking than the first twelve weeks—that's why we are all so cautious and afraid to lift a finger or even tell our family or friends until we make it through twelve weeks and breathe a big sigh of relief. Around this time, some women see their waistline thicken, but most athletes have a strong core and abdomen. You may not show at all until the second trimester, espe-cially if this is your first pregnancy. They say that repeat moms show earlier in subsequent pregnancies, even if their core is strong (prob-ably because the uterus itself is a bit stretched out). Every person's body is different and will show pregnancy a bit differently.

But even if you are not showing, people who know you well may have guessed your condition. They look at you and ask them-selves: Not drinking? Check. Mysteriously bigger boobs? Check. Running to the rest-room before, after, and sometimes during meetings or workouts? Check. Wanting to be home by 7 p.m. on the weekends? Fall-ing asleep in movies, even suspenseful ones? Check! Check! Check! Experienced moms will recognize some of your less obvious com-plaints, too. Is your nose stuffed up all the time? That's estrogen at work again, making the mucous membranes swell—it's so com-mon it's even got a name: pregnancy rhinitis. Are you burping a lot? Get used to it, your mom friends will tell you. And about the best thing we can say about morning sickness, if you've been suffering with it, is that those symptoms subside for almost all women by the fourth month, so hang in there!

Toward the end of the first trimester, the hormone relaxin really goes to work as it builds to its peak output at about fourteen weeks. As its name suggests, relaxin relaxes smooth muscle and connective tissue every-where in your body, even places you wouldn't expect, such as your blood vessels and diges-tive tract. It contributes to widening of the pelvis and softening of the cervix in prepa-ration for birth. For more on relaxin and its effects on your body—and workouts!—see Dr. Heller's info on page 63.

THAT BREATHLESS FEELING

Do you feel short of breath? Most pregnant women do, even just going up a flight of stairs, so you might be surprised to learn that your lung function actually improves during pregnancy. You are getting more oxygen

> "At three months I did the Charles River 1-mile swim, and I definitely needed about a nine-hour nap afterward! I wasn't showing, and everyone wondered why I was so slow. I told my coworkers at about eighteen weeks and they were surprised. I thought I'd been acting strange, tired, and nauseous, but they never would have guessed. They said, 'But you're still go-ing to swim practice!' and I thought, 'Of course I have been. Why wouldn't I?'"
>
> —KATE, SWIMMER, MOTHER OF ONE

with each breath than you did before you were pregnant! But if that's the case, why do you feel breathless? First, your diaphragm is elevated, leaving you with less reserve vol-ume (air left in your lungs between breaths). Second, because your baby needs lots of oxy-gen, progesterone makes you super sensitive to carbon dioxide in your blood. So between breaths, you may feel winded, like you can't catch your breath. This causes many preg-nant women to "overbreathe," or hyperven-tilate, which improves the mix of oxygen in the bloodstream.

Later in the pregnancy, the growing baby will push up on the diaphragm even more, and you will become more of a chest breather. Your pectorals and upper traps will have to pick up the slack from your di-aphragm, and they may even "complain" about it with a little soreness. By the ninth month, you will be taking in about 40 percent more oxygen with each breath. Even though you don't feel now as if you have "extra oxy-

CHECKUP WITH DR. HELLER

Two hormones, estrogen and relaxin, drive most of the changes in your body during pregnancy. Estrogen propels the growth processes and relaxin helps your body prepare for pregnancy and delivery. It's not just the baby that is growing. Your uterus, your breasts, your circulatory system, even your mucous membranes are growing as well. The increased blood flow can make your skin itchy and enlarge and soften your mucous membranes, leading to the common stuffy nose known to physicians as pregnancy rhinitis.

The hormone relaxin, produced in greatly increased amounts during pregnancy, lets the muscles and ligaments in the pelvic region relax, allowing the baby to pass through the birth canal. But its effect isn't limited to that one area. For many women, relaxin loosens the whole musculoskeletal system, not just the all-important pelvic girdle. In addition, relaxin causes nonskeletal round muscles to relax, and that includes arteries, veins, and many muscles in the digestive tract. The results? Back pain, low blood pressure, and indigestion!

By the end of the first trimester, women who might be genetically prone to that laxity of ligaments come to me with a number of complaints. The symphysis pubis (the pelvic joint—cartilage joining the pubic bones) and sacroiliac joint can become unstable or even separate slightly, causing pain or at least uncomfortable sensations. The joint between the pelvis and the spine is a really common place for people to get pain. A lot of times women get symptoms related to the spine—lordosis (inward curve of the lumbar region, or swayback) and compensatory kyphosis (rounding of the upper back), depending on how they're carrying their baby. The most common complaints are lower back pain from change of posture, or the joint slipping out of place a little bit, or sciatica. Women who haven't really been working on their musculature are prone to those changes.

But women who have good strength training are less likely to have these problems. To minimize the musculoskeletal effects of relaxin, don't focus exclusively on one sport or activity. Be sure to round out your workouts by incorporating strength drills into your routine. Strengthening your core and lower back now will pay off a lot later in your pregnancy. Just don't lift too much weight, because women who lift too much weight can be susceptible to lower back strains.

gen," the benefits of this for your postpartum workouts are pretty obvious. This is why it will be important for you to get back to training as soon as you feel ready so you can reap the benefits of this fantastic physiological change before your ability to bring in more oxygen returns to your prepregnancy level. By the way, scientist aren't sure exactly how long it takes for that to happen—the effect lingers longer for some women than others.

KEEP AN EYE ON YOUR DIET

When you are pregnant, your blood sugar can fall during and after exercise, and this can make you feel lightheaded. Besides the obvious reason that pregnancy takes energy—the growth of your baby and your own body—your system processes carbohydrates differently in pregnancy. Your body relies more on fat for energy, but the baby demands glucose for its growth. Glucose is "short-term" food, and there is less glucose available for the baby during exercise and (even when you are resting) if you don't eat often enough. So remember to graze. Keep your energy up by eating small quantities of complex carbohydrates frequently—such as fruits, oatmeal, or whole-grain crackers—every three hours plus a bedtime snack.

> "The first trimester was hard, because I had to train myself to take it easy. I often felt best when I was at the gym in the middle of a workout, so I had to remind myself to ease up—now wasn't the time to go for broke."
>
> —JENNA, CROSSFITTER, MOTHER OF ONE

Starting at the end of the first trimester, you need about 300 additional calories a day to support the baby's growth and the 3 to 4 pounds you should be adding each month. If you were maintaining your weight with exercise before, take in an additional 300 calories per day. And as much as we'd like to take those in M&M's, your baby will thank you if you add healthy, nutrient-packed foods.

TIP: HEARTBURN AND HOW TO AVOID IT

Almost all pregnant women suffer from indigestion and heartburn brought on by the relaxation of the circular muscle around the esophagus (another thing you can blame on relaxin!). You probably can't escape it altogether, but you can minimize it by taking these precautions:

- Keep your weight where it should be. Don't gain more than is recommended.
- Wear loose clothing around your waist.
- Graze—eat six small meals, not three big ones.
- Eat slowly; eating fast and gulping makes you swallow more air.
- Stay upright for a couple of hours after you eat and especially don't go to bed on a full stomach.
- Everyone has different "trigger foods," but spicy foods and vegetables in the cabbage family are notorious for causing heartburn. Avoid any foods that cause problems for you (hot sauce was a killer for me). Also avoid peppermint (a classic GERD trigger).
- Sleep with your head elevated on a wedge or a couple of pillows.

RACE DAY REPORT, JUNE 19, 2010

Here I was, three months pregnant with my second child, in my wetsuit with a little baby bump and ready to race the Minuteman Sprint Triathlon (swim 0.25 mile/bike 15 miles/run 4 miles). The air was calm and cool; it was a perfect day for a race. I was unusually calm and enjoying the moment as my swim wave (women 35+) was called over to cross the starting mats and make our way into the water. I could be calm because I put no pressure on myself to try to "win" or even to think that I could win. I thought, "I am racing as a pregnant athlete and just want to enjoy what I am able to accomplish and get it done." I started out strong and maintained a really good pace, maneuvering past people and being careful not to get close to avoid getting kicked in the belly. I made it safely out of the swim and hustled up to the transition area as I stripped off my wetsuit. My transition was quick and flawless as I headed out on the bike. I was pushing hard on the bike and maintained an 85 to 90 rpm, being careful not to kill the legs for the run. I pulled back into the transition area for a smooth dismount and quick T-time, threw on my visor and off on the run I went. My only thought was: make it to the first aid station and swig some Gatorade, splash my head with some water and mile one is done—only three more miles to go! I wasn't sure of my pace because I didn't wear my GPS—no need to obsess over something I couldn't control. I felt so strong—it was an amazing feeling, finishing that race as strong as I did. I was on cloud nine. I never expected the race to go so smoothly.

We've looked at what not to eat; now here's an overview of what you *should* eat every day. Besides your daily prenatal and fish oil/omega-3 supplements, these are the kinds of foods you should put on your menu every day. Pick from the whole list; don't just get stuck on a few favorites, and remember to spread your food intake out in small meals through the day. As you will see, grains (complex carbs) are a significant part of the diet. If you are following a Paleo diet or have wheat allergies or other restrictions, be sure to work with your medical team or speak with a dietician (preferably one who knows about the meal plan you are follow-

ing). They will help you develop a healthy eating plan that fits your dietary interests or restrictions.

- 6 to 11 servings of whole grains (a slice or an ounce) and legumes (½ cup): brown rice, wild rice, whole-grain bread, cereal, or pasta, beans, lentils, peanuts, peas
- 4 to 6 servings of vegetables of all kinds (1 cup raw, ½ cup cooked): winter squash, spinach, kale, lettuce, broccoli, red bell pepper, carrots, sweet potato, green beans, zucchini, mushrooms, corn, broccoli, cauliflower, tomatoes

- 3 to 5 servings of fruits (one medium fruit or ½ cup chunks): orange, grapefruit, kiwi, berries, mango, peach, papaya, melon, avocado, apricot, apple, pear, banana, cherries
- 3 to 5 servings of dairy or other calcium sources (1 cup milk, ½ cup other sources): milk, hard cheese, yogurt, collard greens, edamame, sesame seeds, calcium-fortified juice, canned salmon with bones, tofu

- 3 to 5 servings of protein and iron sources (2–3 ounces): meat, poultry, fish, eggs, nuts, cheese, yogurt, peanut butter, tofu, edamame, sardines, spinach, dried fruit, beans, soy products, seeds
- 4 servings of fats (1–2 tablespoons): peanut butter, avocado, sour cream, cream cheese, cream, salad dressing, oil, butter, mayonnaise
- 8 (8-ounce) glasses of water

THE TRAINING EFFECT OF PREGNANCY

Research shows that exercising through pregnancy and after has a training effect that is greater than what nonpregnant women can achieve over the same time period. In fact, the effect is so marked that in the 1980s some Eastern European Olympic athletes were accused of getting pregnant just for the benefits it confers!

The data show that women who train through pregnancy increase their aerobic capacity by about 10 percent, even if their training volume declines a bit. Blood volume increases by about 60 percent, which mimics the effects of doping. Not surprisingly, mothers report that they have improved focus and mental attitude, and greatly increased ability to tolerate pain—all useful tools for a competitor!

Paula Radcliffe is a case in point; she trained through her 2006 pregnancy, even running the day before labor, then won the 2007 New York Marathon and delivering. And remember, there is some data that supports the ability of a pregnant woman to increase her strength during pregnancy as well. Your time to fatigue may come sooner; however, your short burst of energy—during low-rep strength training with ample rest between sets—is not compromised. Although you may not be able to increase or work at your VO2Max (a measure of how efficient your body is at using its oxygen supply) during your pregnancy, you do have the capacity to increase some of your more stable joint lifts such as front and back squats and deadlifts.

Steve

> ### OLD WIVES' TALE: EXERCISING THROUGH PREGNANCY INTERFERES WITH THE BABY'S GROWTH.
>
> Studies conducted by James F. Clapp, MD, show that sustained, intense exercise during pregnancy affects only one aspect of fetal growth: fat. Babies born to exercising mothers tend to be thinner, but not low birth weight. Their head, organs, and development are all normal—they are just less fat.
>
> Far from endangering the baby, by improving blood supply to the placenta regular exercise improves the baby's ability to deal with the intermittent reductions in uterine blood flow and oxygen delivery that are a part of everyday life. This could prove very valuable in the case of a traumatic injury or a medical emergency.

TO COMPETE OR NOT TO COMPETE?

When I found out I was pregnant the first time, racing was the last thing on my mind. I had been advised to keep my heart rate low and hadn't yet learned to ignore that old wives' tale. But as the weeks went by I felt so good that I couldn't resist keeping up my training enough to complete the Philadelphia half marathon in November, the end of my first trimester. Some people thought I was crazy running a half marathon at three months, but I knew that Joan Benoit Samuelson had actually completed the 1987 Boston Marathon when she was three months pregnant. I decided to take it easy with a low-key approach to keep from pushing myself too hard before I got my doctor's approval. So I trained and ran it easy, enjoying the company of my best friend who kept me at a nice comfortable pace. If you have any concerns about your exercise program during your pregnancy, this is a good approach: train easy and maintain your fitness until you have a chance to talk things over with your doctor. Bear in mind that the actual event is less stressful than the months of training to peak for it.

On the other hand, you may want to compete, as I did during my second pregnancy. Under the guidance of my trainer, my ob/gyn, and Steve, I was following my coach's plan to prepare for the Minuteman Sprint Triathlon at the end of my third month. Some days I felt strong and enjoyed the training; other days I felt PREGNANT! I had many moments when I thought "Why?!" But when I pushed through those days and the negative feelings, I would have a great workout and then feel amazing the next few days. I never let my negative thoughts keep me from working out, but if I wasn't feeling up to doing hill repeats I would just do a few and then finish with a lower intensity run. Some days that was challenging enough. My toughest week was right before the race. No matter what I did, I just felt slow, uncomfortable and pregnant. This wasn't helping me feel good about the race coming up, but I stayed focused and didn't worry.

A BIG MILESTONE: SEEING THE DOCTOR

For normal, healthy pregnancies, many doctors encourage the first prenatal visit in the third month. You probably will be relieved to finally get the official go-ahead from your physician (assuming you have found a doctor who will support your efforts). Now is a good time to frankly discuss your current program and which activities you hope to keep up during your pregnancy, assuming all systems remain "go." If your doctor has worked with other pregnant athletes, she

---

THE PROS

Named both Rookie of the Year and Most Valuable Player for the 2008 WNBA season, star Candace Parker announced her pregnancy in January 2009. After the birth of her daughter, she missed the first eight games of the 2009 season. Several high-profile college basketball players have competed right through their pregnancies, concealing their condition with surprising ease and playing amazingly. Florida A&M's guard Tameka McKelton played well into the 2010–2011 season. "I basically just gritted my teeth, went to practice every morning even though I was sick, flew on the planes, and just played as hard as I could, but carefully," she told reporters.

"The big thing we've discovered is that athletes can feel like they have to hide it, for fear of losing their scholarship," said Steve Walz, assistant athletic director for sports medicine at the University of San Francisco. The NCAA passed legislation to assure that a woman's scholarship isn't reduced because of pregnancy, partially prompted by media reports and recent examples of women concealing pregnancies including:

- Fantasia Goodwin (Syracuse) told her coach the night before the last game of the season. He held her out of that game and she delivered her daughter two months later.
- Connie Neal (Louisville) played eleven games in 2003 (up to eight months pregnant) before finally telling coaches. Her last game was December 20 and she gave birth to her daughter January 31. She returned to practice four weeks later and played the end of the season.
- USF guard Rae Rae Sayles played five games in 2003 before it was learned she was pregnant; after taking a year off, she left the team to focus on her daughter.

With proper supervision and care from doctors, athletes can safely participate in college athletics in the early stages of pregnancy. Elizabeth Sorensen, assistant professor at the College of Nursing and Health and NCAA faculty athletics representative at Wright State Ohio, said research shows that in the first fourteen weeks of pregnancy, a fetus is so small and still protected by a mother's pelvic bones that the risk of injury to mother or child is minimal.

may be able to share some tips from their experiences.

Three months into my first pregnancy, what I heard at our initial appointment with Dr. Heller was music to my ears! After checking the baby and me carefully and listening to my concerns and aspirations, he gave me the news that changed my whole approach and led to this book: "Keep up with the fitness program. Don't worry about your heart rate, but do pay attention to your perceived exertion." Dr. Heller told me to listen to my body and keep doing what I had been doing. And that's exactly what I did for the remainder of that pregnancy and all through the second one. I continued intensive workouts, resting when fatigued and modifying my routine from month to month and then week to week as my body changed. Here's what I was up to in Month 3 of my second pregnancy.

WHAT ABOUT "ENERGY PRODUCTS"?

Especially if you are an endurance athlete, you may use gels, sports drinks, or other performance foods on long runs or swims. But be cautious about using them through pregnancy. Read the labels—many of these supplements contain massive doses of caffeine and sugar, which will send your blood sugar on a roller-coaster ride. Even more concerning, they may contain supplements that have not been tested on pregnant women. While energy bars and gels are handy and easier to carry than the foods they replace, they may not be any better at giving you a burst of energy. A handful of raisins or a banana might be a better choice.

Sunday	Monday	Tuesday	Wednesday	Thursday	Friday	Saturday
Off or easy swim	Morning run, strength; evening bike	Morning boot camp run; evening swim	Morning bike, strength; evening short run	Morning track run; evening swim	Morning bike, strength	Morning strength, swim, bike, and/or run (a brick workout)

MY MONTH 3
STRENGTH WORKOUT

Suggested modifications for Month 3: If you are still having issues with nausea or lightheadedness, take it a little easier or time your workouts for the time of day when you feel best. Don't add unaccustomed heavy weight to squats. Put your hands under your butt for any leg lifts to protect your lower back. Otherwise, you should have no problem completing these routines, no matter what your sport or preferred activity.

If you swim more than 30 minutes or so, have a light snack a half-hour or so beforehand, drink plenty of fluids during the session and have some glucose to keep the blood sugar levels up. The glucose can be in a liquid (Gatorade, G2, PowerAde, etc.) or in solid form (Gu gels, jelly beans, and gummy bears). If you already have a child—especially if he or she is over four years old—you probably have enough of these little sugary snacks in the cracks of your car seats to help refuel for any athletic event.

If your sport is one that requires sudden bursts of intensity, such as soccer or basketball, pay attention to your sprints and be sure to recover after dashing down the field or court. Don't let your heart rate stay at its maximum for more than a moment, and pay attention when you decelerate and change direction. It is during these points within your movement that you are most likely to be injured, so be mindful of your limits and the intensity you put into it.

The Workout

Equipment needed: Physioball/bench; Bosu ball; ankle bands; barbell or dumbbells

Dynamic Warm-up: Refer to page 15 for the full Dynamic Warm-up.

Conditioning Circuit #1 (1 exercise): Complete this 2 times with 30-second rest between runs.

Exercise #1: Shuttle Run
Reps: 15-yard shuttle run 4 times

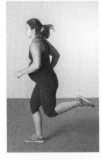

SHUTTLE RUN

Strength Circuit (6 exercises): Complete this circuit 3 times.

Exercise #1: Overhead Plate Hold Forward Lunge Walk (Lunge focus)

Reps: 25-yard lunge walk

Exercise #2: Dumbbell Plank Rows (Core and Pull focus)

Reps: 10 alternating plank rows per arm

Exercise #3: Deadlifts (use dumbbells or barbell) (Bend/Hip Flexion focus)

Reps: 20

Exercise #4: Bosu Lateral Lunge (weight optional) (Lunge focus)

Reps: 15 per side

Exercise #5: Ankle Band Lateral Shuffle (Push focus)

Reps: 25 yards per lead leg

Exercise #6: Physioball Walkout w/Push-up and Double-leg Knee Tuck (Core and Push focus)

Reps: 15

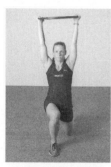

OVERHEAD PLATE HOLD FORWARD LUNGE WALK

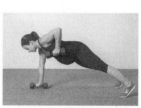

DUMBBELL PLANK ROWS

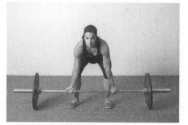

DEADLIFTS

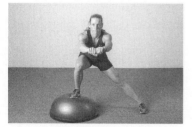

BOSU LATERAL LUNGE

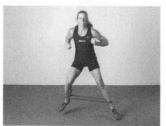

ANKLE BAND LATERAL SHUFFLE

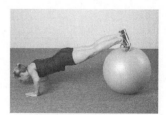

PHYSIOBALL WALKOUT W/PUSH-UP AND DOUBLE-LEG KNEE TUCK

Metabolic Circuit: Barbell Burpee Jump-overs w/Sprint

Reps: 5-Minute AMRAP (as many repetitions as possible) of 5 burpees followed by a 30-yard sprint.

Cool Down and Stretch:

Static stretch, mobility work, foam roller: Follow the Stretch Routine introduced on page 18.

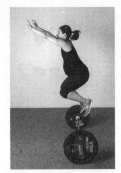

**BARBELL BURPEE
JUMP-OVERS W/SPRINT**

Believe Me,
I'm Pregnant!

Your Body Now

Strength	You're strong; keep it that way by avoiding overstressing your pelvic area.
Agility	If you have a bump, it is too small to affect your balance yet.
Stamina	Even if you feel winded, you can probably push through.
Well-being	Most women feel great in the second trimester, although you may have some mood swings or difficulty concentrating. If you have headaches, take acetaminophen (Tylenol), not aspirin.
Nutrition	Morning sickness should abate, allowing you to fuel your workouts and the baby's growth by returning to your prepregnancy caloric intake or slightly more. Keep grazing to minimize lightheadedness and heartburn.
Modifications	Don't lie on your belly if you have a bump and it makes you uncomfortable. Buy a larger bra.
Your baby now	By the fourth month, the baby is about as big as an onion, 4½ inches from head to butt, and weighs about 6 ounces; the heartbeat is audible.

By now you have noticed some weight gain. The baby itself still weighs less than half a pound, but most women add 2 to 4 pounds in the first trimester. Your body is adding blood volume and building tissues (think: breasts) to support the baby. "Eating for two" means eating wisely, but let's face it:

pregnancy does funny things to us hormonally. Nobody's perfect and I was no nutrition angel myself. I indulged in the occasional raspberry bismarck, which I would *never* do when in race mode except as a treat after an event! Just choose your treats carefully. One of the biggest reasons I wanted to keep

---

**OLD WIVES' TALE:
IF YOU DON'T EAT WHAT YOU ARE CRAVING, THE BABY WILL BE BORN
WITH A BIRTHMARK IN THE SHAPE OF THE FOOD YOU DESIRE.**

This might be an excellent way to get your partner out at midnight to pick up that pint of Chunky Monkey, so it will be our little secret that it is—of course—totally unfounded in fact.

---

up with my training was so I could have ice cream and not regret it!

You may be starting to show a little, and sporting your "baby bump" now. The bump will be noticeable only to your friends and family unless you are wearing tight clothes. The size of your bump is one of the factors that will influence your workouts, because as the bump grows, your balance and center of gravity change and you start to feel that you are squishing your baby when you lie face-down. This shouldn't be a problem yet, but as you notice these changes in the coming weeks, make adjustments in your routine. On the plus side, your breasts are less tender, although they continue to grow. Buy a new sports bra if you've outgrown your old one. Don't buy too many at once—you'll need a larger size before too long. But don't buy large and plan to "grow into it," either—you want it to be tight enough to support you, but not strangling.

Your energy is good. Most women feel less fatigued after the first trimester is over. In fact, some women say they never felt as good or as full of energy as they did in mid-pregnancy! Honestly, the toughest part of Month 4 is the transition from a more ath-letic, lean body into a body that's obviously carrying a baby. You might find it hard to get used to a bulge around your middle, but this is what a healthy pregnancy looks like, and your goal is a healthy baby.

The reason you are starting to show is that the position of the uterus changes as the baby grows. Around Month 4 or early in Month 5, the uterus rises above the pelvic rim and displaces the intestine, giving you a little paunch as the baby begins to move up and out (and you ain't seen nothin' yet!). Your bump will seem to grow every day, and there's not much you can do about its size. If you are short it may really "pop," as the baby only has one direction to go: out! Besides the baby's new visibility, this new position affects your internal organs, too. There is less pressure on your bladder, so you may notice that you make fewer trips to the bathroom. Enjoy it while you can!

You may notice that you seem to get out of breath even more than you did last month. As the baby moves upward, it presses on your diaphragm, diminishing your lung capacity and leaving less air in your lungs after you exhale (this is called reserve volume). So, be-tween breaths, women sometimes feel more

CHECKUP WITH DR. HELLER: TESTS, TESTS, AND MORE TESTS

The fourth month is when you start to get the results of the standard tests. Most women want to know about the ultrasound, find out the baby's gender, and review the results of any screenings for diseases and conditions. This is always an athlete's most nerve-racking time at the doctor's office—until you learn that your baby is healthy and you can continue to work out. There are a couple of findings at this time that might lead your medical team to recommend that you change your activity.

Besides often informing you of your baby's gender, the ultrasound will identify the position of the placenta. Placenta previa is a condition in which the placenta grows in the lowest part of the uterus, covering the cervix. Some providers might suggest "pelvic rest" in this case—stopping intercourse because penetration could cause bleeding. A few will suggest decreasing exercise, and this is more likely if their patient has experienced some vaginal bleeding.

Sometimes the ultrasound is the first indication that the woman is expecting twins (or more!). With the larger uterus, the woman's center of gravity is thrown off earlier than it would be with a single birth, so modifications should be made in any activity that requires balance, such as single-leg exercises. Morning sickness tends to linger longer in the pregnancies of twins, so you might not feel up to exercising too strenuously. Most seriously, multiple births carry an increased risk of preterm labor. In the second half of the pregnancy, the larger uterus extends and exerts pressure on the cervix—the pressure is both greater and earlier than normal because the uterus is bearing the weight of two babies. Gravity and repeated impact can cause the cervix to shorten and dilate early, leading to preterm delivery. At around eighteen weeks, the medical team will begin to measure cervical length. If it is shortened, this will probably lead to a recommendation of diminished activity or even work restrictions.

Another routine test you'll undergo a little later (between Weeks 24 and 28) is a glucose screening, which will indicate whether further testing for gestational diabetes is necessary. While very rare in women who have a long-standing history of regular exercise, gestational diabetes can be dangerous if left untreated. Luckily, diet and exercise go a long way toward controlling it.

winded, as if they can't catch their breath as easily. This has two main causes. First, your uterus is pressing on your diaphragm: Less room, less air left in the lungs between breaths. The second factor is the effect of the hormone progesterone, which essentially tricks your brain, causing you to feel winded constantly. There's a huge spectrum in how much this affects pregnant women. But most women notice that they are breathing harder at the same level of exertion as the months go on. This is normal—you will naturally adjust your activity level if you are attentive to your perceived exertion. Meanwhile, when was the last time you felt winded just walking up a flight of stairs? Well, get used to that!

Now that the baby's position is changing, it's time to develop new sleep habits. If you usually sleep on your back or facedown, learn to sleep on your left side now. Lying on your back or stomach later in pregnancy decreases blood circulation to the baby; sleeping on the left side provides the best blood flow to the baby because it keeps the weight of your bowel and other organs off the uterus and the veins returning blood to your heart. Practice falling asleep on your left side and if you wake up in the night (make that *when* you wake up in the night!) return to this position to go back to sleep. Don't worry if you wake up on your back or belly; just turn over onto your side. If anything were really wrong, your body will certainly be able to wake up and take care of the issue.

FOOD, GLORIOUS FOOD

If you've been suffering from morning sickness, you can most likely kiss that problem good-bye in the fourth month. Your appetite will start to increase and you will begin to enjoy eating again. Now you can begin to slowly add calories to support the two growth processes that are under way—the baby's and yours. But just because morning sickness is a thing of the past doesn't mean that the digestive effects of pregnancy are be-

> "Thank God I could work out. If I wasn't allowed that physical outlet, I feel like bad things would happen, particularly to the people around me! It brings my whole ecosystem into balance."
>
> —CAROL, TRIATHLETE, MOTHER OF TWO

hind you. You may continue to experience some food cravings and aversions (increased estrogen heightens your sense of smell), although these usually taper off by the end of the month. This is another example of how each pregnancy is unique—my experiences in two pregnancies were completely different. Eating was challenging throughout my first pregnancy. After making it through evening sickness in the first trimester, I had some food aversions that hung around for the whole nine months. Even though chicken had been a big staple in my diet, just the thought of it made me nauseous. Right after I gave birth, I could enjoy chicken again. Weird. My second pregnancy was totally different and great as far as my diet was concerned.

EATING FOR TWO: I'VE GOT A CRAVING . . .

The stereotypical "pregnant lady" cravings are pickles and ice cream, but you may have found yourself with an unreasonable desire for something else. About half of pregnant women report at least one craving—ranging from the very sweet to the very salty. Remember those hormonal changes that made you so sensitive to smell in the morning sickness days? They're still at work, and that increase in estrogen may be responsible for any cravings and food aversions you're experiencing.

Pay attention to your cravings but don't be snookered by them. Indulge the healthy ones and try to find yourself an acceptable alternative for that second jelly doughnut; if you must succumb, limit yourself to *one* brownie, not an entire batch. Eat frequent small meals to keep your blood sugar stable, and (of course) get your exercise.

Rarely, a craving may signal a deficiency. If you get a hankering for clay, ashes, or any other really strange things, call your doctor, who will check your iron. But if you are care-ful about your nutrition there's no need to give in to every craving. After all, as author Elizabeth Somer says, "If people craved what the body needs, we would all eat more broc-coli and less chocolate."

OTHER ALIMENTARY DELIGHTS

As if heartburn wasn't enough, now you'll have constipation to deal with, too! Relaxin is doing its job on the muscles of the bowel, causing nutrients to linger longer for better absorption. And, in your internal real estate as in everything else, the baby gets first dibs; as the baby's position changes, your bowel gets the squeeze. Luckily, the solution for

---

TIP: YOUR ACHING MUSCLES

You're familiar with DOMS (delayed onset muscle soreness), but now that you are pregnant you can't just pop an aspirin or an ibuprofen to relieve aches and pains. Turn instead to RICE:

- Rest the affected area.
- Ice it. I like to freeze paper cups full of water and roll them on the sore spots.
- Compression. Wrap in an elastic bandage.
- Elevation.

You might also consider having a massage. Some massage therapists are certified in pre-natal massage; many use special tables with hollowed-out areas for your belly and breasts, or will massage you while you lie on your side. If you've been accustomed to acupuncture treatments, you can continue them.

You may be used to training every day or maybe only having one day of recovery. But when you are pregnant and training hard, be smart and don't work through extreme soreness. If you are really sore the next day, take it off from exercise and add more stretching sessions in. It's okay to train through regular or mild stiff muscles, but when you can barely walk, you need to stop for a day or two.

constipation is the same as for heartburn and lightheadedness: small, frequent meals of complex carbohydrates (think: fiber!) and plenty of hydration (prune juice is a liquid, too). Oh, and did I mention exercise? We all know how exercise keeps things moving.

A related issue that you may have to deal with is hemorrhoids. These are actually varicose veins (which may also pop up on your legs when you're pregnant) brought on by the pressure of the uterus on the rectum and exacerbated by constipation. They hurt, they itch, they bleed—they are the original "pain in the ass." Avoiding constipation helps, so take in plenty of fiber and fluids. Keep moving—prolonged standing and sitting increase pressure on the "affected area." Oh, and did I mention exercise? Your usual workouts will help keep you "regular," and Kegels will increase blood circulation in the pelvic floor (for a how-to on Kegels, see page 89).

'SNOT A PROBLEM

Your mucous membranes are yet another target of estrogen and progesterone. Increased blood flow may give you a stuffy nose and ears. Check with your medical practitioner before you take any medicine, but you can relieve these symptoms with some old-fashioned remedies: taking steamy showers, using a humidifier, and elevating your head to sleep (a twofer: also a good fix for heartburn). Did I mention exercise and

As Brandi was beginning to show, the realization that we were having a child and that our first child was *inside my wife* really hit home, and the nerves kicked in a bit. Boy, was our life about to change! I also really began to appreciate all the hard work she had been doing (workouts in particular) and continued to do for the full term of the pregnancy. In the first pregnancy, once her belly popped a bit I started being more mindful of how she was training (even though other people at the gym hadn't even figured out she was pregnant!). We learned so much during that first pregnancy, so the second time around I was more comfortable and could wholeheartedly encourage her exercise routines. I was so excited to see her keep up her intensity and exercise regimen. She didn't seem to miss a beat in regard to her lifting and triathlon training—she was a true inspiration to me. But we did have to laugh that many people thought she was a bit off her rocker! As long as the doctor visits kept confirming how well the pregnancy was going and how healthy she was, there was no slowing down for her as far as I was concerned, even though my enthusiasm created some friction and humor between us as the months progressed!

Steve

hydrating? Both will help the body rid itself of excess fluids.

It's also pretty common for your gums to bleed after you brush or floss, for the same reason—increased blood flow to the mucous membranes. But don't let this make you avoid flossing and regular brushing with a soft brush, because your gums are extra vulnerable to bacteria now. Visit your dentist for your regular checkup (remember to tell him or her you're pregnant).

I AM *NOT* CRANKY!

If you (or your partner) hoped that pregnancy would bring a break from the premenstrual moodiness that some women experience, think again. And it's no wonder you're on an emotional roller coaster. You're dealing with a double whammy: the same hormones that trigger PMS symptoms combine with the stress of upcoming parenthood to make you irritable and maybe give you a bit of a hair trigger. Face it, there's a lot going on. Your body is changing every day, and not always for the better, despite all your efforts. The list of the pregnancy dos and don'ts would be daunting even if you could focus, which you probably can't. And you may not be getting enough sleep either, with heartburn or anxious thoughts cutting into your zzzs. Knowing where all this moodiness comes from may help you (and your partner) cut yourself some slack.

One thing you can do is keep a positive attitude. There are some great books out there that will tell you exactly what is going

"It's great for my students to see me go through this process. They are aspiring dance professionals—performers and teachers—and they need to see that it's okay. When I was demonstrating a tricky combination, one of them said, 'Oh my God, she dances better than me!' That felt good."

—MEGHAN, DANCER, MOTHER OF ONE

on during each month and how the baby is growing, but I chose not to read anything that would make me nervous or afraid to continue exercise. With all the emotional intensity of pregnancy, I didn't want to get caught up in the "what ifs" of any and every little thing I did. If you find yourself having second thoughts or doubting yourself, talk to your doctor and your partner. Also remember to give yourself a break and trust in the fact that the human race is very resilient.

TAKING THE PLUNGE

One thing I did to test this notion of resiliency was participate in national "Polar Plunge" day when I was four months pregnant with Mackenzie. I had done this plunge for several years, but this time, of course, what had been a simple trot into the ocean was different, even though on New Year's Day north of Boston, the ocean is warmer than the air! I decided to wear my heart rate monitor just to keep an eye on things. During the plunge, my heart rate jumped to about 170 (a normal range for

---

PEOPLE SAY THE MOST AMAZING THINGS . . .

"Take it easy!" How many times a day do you hear that? Or how's this for a confidence booster: "Are you sure you aren't hurting the baby?" This is one of the first old wives' tales that I had to discuss with Dr. Heller.

If you have been working out for a long time, your family will know how important it is to you. Like Sarah, whose partner said, "As long as the doctor is okay with it, I am okay with it," or Ashley, who told me, "My husband knows better than to tell me what to do," you will come to an understanding.

But sometimes even perfect strangers feel free to comment on how you look and what you are doing, and this goes double if you are working out! Most people were incredibly supportive, cheering me on at races and keeping track of my progress at the gym. But what to say to folks who feel obliged to share their unsupportive or even negative thoughts?

- Say nothing. It's always an option to just keep moving.
- Tell the truth. "My doctor is aware of my training and supports me in what I am doing."
- Go for the teachable moment. "Do you know that the American College of Obstetrics and Gynecology encourages exercise during pregnancy and supports women continuing doing their usual fitness activities as long as they feel up to it? I feel great, by the way!"
- Try humor. "Ha! This is nothing! Did you hear about the lady who ran the Chicago Marathon and then ran straight to the hospital to give birth!?"
- Go on the offensive. "Looks like you could use a little jog yourself—care to join me?"

---

me during exercise). I've since heard from several experienced open water swimmers who swam through their pregnancies. They didn't shock their bodies like I did with a big New Year's Day surprise, but acclimated to the dropping water temperature with regular swims throughout the year—probably a much better idea!

If you have made your pregnancy public, you are surely beginning to get lots of advice, some of it questioning your decision to maintain your fitness, some of it questioning your sanity! You'll find tips for responding to comments in the box above. Your belly should still be pretty flat except for that little bump, so you can still accomplish the rigorous routine included in this chapter (if your bump protrudes more, be sure to modify accordingly). Don't be alarmed if you seem to perspire more—that is your thyroid at work. You'll also be breathing pretty hard because of the upward pressure on your diaphragm, adding to the hormonal effects we discussed last month.

This month will be a big transition for you mentally. Stay strong and passionate about what you are doing and try not to let the discomfort of your changing body keep you from doing what you do. You're used to listening to your body and will know when you need to start modifying workouts and intensity levels from here on out. The first four months were nothing compared to what the next five months will bring. I was able to keep up my schedule, even if the intensity was changing.

Sunday	Monday	Tuesday	Wednesday	Thursday	Friday	Saturday
Off or easy swim	Morning run, strength; evening bike	Morning boot camp run; evening swim	Morning bike, strength; evening short run	Morning track run; evening swim	Morning bike, strength	Morning strength, swim, bike, and/or run (a brick workout)

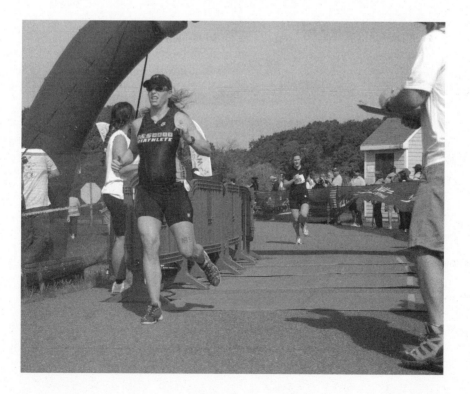

MONTH 4
STRENGTH WORKOUT

Suggested modifications: You may be feeling pretty good in Month 4, with nausea a thing of the past. If you have a small bump it will not really affect your balance yet. But pay attention to your body and notice the difference between something just being "hard" and something that makes you uncomfortable. For example, you may not be comfortable lying on your belly, so say goodbye to exercises in the prone position, such as Superman extensions, until you deliver your baby.

If you swim in open water, remember to be alert to hypothermia. Your core will stay warm, but your hands and feet may get cold. If you can't pull your fingers together or you get lightheaded, get out and warm up! If you swim in the pool, you may find flip turns give you reflux and an acid feeling in your mouth. As is the case with heartburn, progestogen has relaxed the sphincter at the end of the esophagus.

If you are a runner, consider altering your route or reducing the frequency of your runs. As relaxin starts to affect your joints, the crown of the road, or the off-road running trails you have frequented these past weeks (months, years, etc.!), may now be putting your lower limb joints at risk of injury. As relaxin takes its toll, be aware that the more unstable or angled the surface (crowned streets), the more likely it is to strain those joints and ligaments. To reduce this danger, do your best to run on flat surfaces or, if you are running on the road, run equal time on each side of the road if possible.

If you are expecting multiples, you are probably beginning to feel it! Monitor your fatigue and rest when you are tired. Support your belly with a band or belt. Continue to be mindful of how you are feeling—although you may be in the earlier stages of pregnancy, your body is further along as far as the size of the baby goes. You may have to deal with changes you would not have had to manage until later months if you were only carrying one child. Therefore, take steps to continue to be active, but consider doing fewer and fewer single-leg exercises. Decrease or eliminate any jumping or explosive exercises as well as very heavy single- or low-rep exercises where you put additional internal pressure on the pelvic floor.

If you are weight training, be sure to warm up well. Train with moderate weights but high repetitions.

The Workout

Equipment needed: Barbell; sled; plyo box; medicine ball; physioball; dumbell; rings/TRX

Dynamic Warm-up (see page 15)

Conditioning Circuit: Complete the circuit 2 times with 2 minutes' rest after each set.
Shuttle Run (200 yards total) > Weighted Drive Sled Push (25 yards out and back)

Strength Circuit (7 exercises): Complete this circuit 3 times

Exercise #1: Barbell Hang Clean (Compound Movement)

Reps: 12

Exercise #2: Box Step-up to Lateral Lunge (Squat and Lunge focus)

Reps: 15 per side

Exercise #3: Side Bridge pulses (Core focus)

Reps: 30 sec per side

Exercise #4: Ring or TRX back rows (Pull focus)

Reps: 20

Exercise #5: Single-leg Romanian Deadlift (Bend focus)

Reps: 15 per side

Exercise #6: Single-arm Dumbbell or Kettlebell Snatch (Compound Movement)

Reps: 10 per side

Exercise #7: Medicine Ball Butterfly Sit-up (Core focus)

Reps: 20

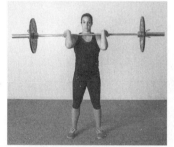

BARBELL HANG CLEAN

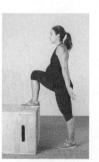

BOX STEP-UP TO LATERAL LUNGE

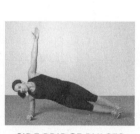

SIDE BRIDGE PULSES

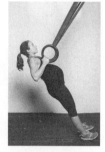

RING OR TRX BACK ROWS

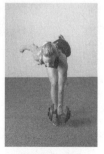

SINGLE-LEG ROMANIAN DEADLIFT

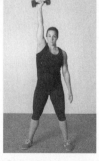

SINGLE-ARM DUMBBELL OR KETTLEBELL SNATCH

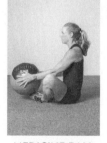

MEDICINE BALL BUTTERFLY SIT-UP

Cool Down and Stretch:

Static stretch, mobility work, foam roller: Follow the Stretch Routine introduced on page 18.

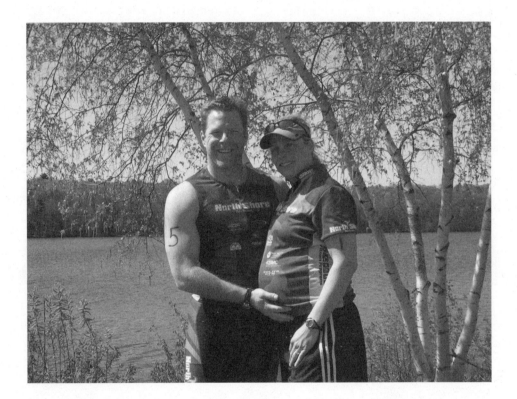

Does This Pregnancy Make Me Look Fat?

Your Body Now

Strength	You can and should continue to build both lower and upper body strength with a focus on your back and posture as the lower back will always seem to be engaged.
Agility	Your balance may be affected by the bump, so be alert if you are doing anything that requires rapid side-to-side movement.
Stamina	You will notice the effects of carrying more weight, even if it's "all baby." You will get very familiar with sucking wind.
Well-being	Most discomforts of pregnancy fade in the second trimester and women tend to feel good in Month 5, with plenty of energy. Moods can range from calm to irritable, with forgetfulness. If leg cramps wake you up, try doing calf raises during the day.
Nutrition	Add 300 calories a day from now until you deliver—or after delivery if you breast-feed.
Modifications	Do not lie on your back for long periods; be careful of hips and lower back. Reassess, modify, or discontinue any activity that makes you feel shaky or off balance.
Your baby now	The baby measures about 10 inches from head to heel and weighs 12 ounces. The toenails and fingernails have started growing.

A month or so ago, people looked at you and wondered, "Is she? . . ." Face it: Those days are gone. By Month 5, you clearly look pregnant and you probably feel pretty bulky.

Even your bumps have bumps! Around Month 5 or 6, your belly button and nipples will pop out, whether they were "innies" or "outies" before. The navel is literally being pushed out by the uterus as it rises and increases in size. The pregnancy hormones are getting your nipples ready for nursing. Your nipples may never return to their original shape, but your belly button will go back to normal soon after delivery.

Your baby weighs less than a pound, but that combined with the placenta and increased uterine muscle will start to make sleeping on your back pretty uncomfortable. Besides interfering with blood flow, sleeping with the whole weight of your pregnancy on your back and intestines is a one-way ticket to backache and hemorrhoids, and it will only get worse from now on. As you've probably already abandoned sleeping on your belly, that leaves your side. The left side is best, because of the locations of various internal organs, especially your bowel (sleeping on the left keeps that weight off the baby). A body pillow is a lifesaver.

You may still experience some faintness and dizziness, but there's a new reason for this now-familiar problem: the pressure of your uterus on the blood vessels that return blood from your lower body. A sudden shift of blood away from the brain, caused by standing or changing position quickly, can make you feel woozy. The solution? Just don't stand up too fast! Take your time returning to an upright position, especially if your head has been below your waist (for inchworms, for instance). Work out next to a door frame or something else you can touch to get your balance. Don't hold your breath during lifts. Finally, avoid having low blood sugar by grazing and eating protein at every meal, and stay well hydrated.

OLD WIVES' TALES: IF YOU HAVE A LOT OF HEARTBURN, YOU WILL HAVE A BABY WITH A LOT OF HAIR.

Given the prevalence of heartburn during pregnancy, it's inevitable that there will be an old wives' tale about it. Amazingly, this one might be true! A 2006 Johns Hopkins University study showed a correlation between heartburn and hairier babies. Turns out that the same high levels of estrogen that relax the esophagus can lead to more fetal hair growth. As the *New York Times* reported (February 20, 2007), the findings came as a shock to Kathleen Costigan, lead author of the study. "We've heard this claim hundreds of times, and I've always told people it's nonsense," she said. "Since the study came out, I've had to eat a lot of crow."

WEIGHING IN

Now that you are well into the second trimester, you should have gained 5 to 10 pounds—if you have not, take a look at your eating habits. Be sure that you are taking in enough calories and timing your meals to support your pregnancy and your workouts. Concentrate on nutrient-rich foods and eat immediately after long, hard workouts (and sometimes during, if they are very long, such as one-hour-plus cardio-based workouts) to make sure that enough food reaches the baby when your body is making extra demands. For example, after a cardio-based or

---

CHECKUP WITH DR. HELLER

Most pregnant women are rightly cautious about taking any kind of medication. But I always advise women to be proactive in addressing heartburn. I've had at least one patient who developed scarring of the esophagus from the recurring reflux common in pregnancy. Chronic acid reflux can lead to permanent damage of the esophagus, causing more difficult and chronic problems, so heartburn is not something anyone should suffer through. Feel free to use a mild antacid, such as Tums or Mylanta, or an H-2 blocker, such as Zantac or Pepcid. Antacids and H-2 blockers (that actually reduce the production of acid) are fine to take throughout the pregnancy. Some people need even more, and I'll suggest Prilosec or something like that. And of course, follow all the behavioral modifications suggested on page 64.

By the way, I do not recommend that pregnant women take any other drugs without consulting their medical practitioners. Athletes may be accustomed to taking ibuprofen or naproxen for muscle aches and strains. These medications are generally to be avoided in pregnancy, but your provider may allow you to take a brief course during certain times of the pregnancy. Acetaminophen is a better choice for pain relief during pregnancy. Antihistamines are generally safe for seasonal allergies. Menthol heat is generally safe. Some decongestants are safe, unless there are concerns regarding blood pressure.

---

strength training–based workout, consider eating a nutrient and carb-rich sweet potato, a great source of complex, lower glycemic carbohydrate that will help replenish your glycogen (sugar) stores without spiking your insulin levels.

If your weight is on track, you can be a little less strict nutritionally. Indulge in the occasional fruit-filled pancake breakfast— why not? After all, you are pregnant and working out—you should be able to treat yourself now and then.

Now is when you really notice your shape changing, and you may feel uncomfortable in your own skin if you are accustomed to a lean, athletic body. Just like any other woman when it comes to the "weigh in," I would remove my jacket, sneakers, or sandals, and anything in my pockets to avoid adding a single extra ounce to that number! But I also knew that my body was adding important support for the baby. By the ninth month, most women put on 3 pounds of blood and 2 pounds of breast tissue. The uterus and placenta add 3½ pounds. Fluids for the mom and baby account for at least 6 pounds. And the mom must put on new muscle and fat to support a healthy pregnancy. All this, and the baby's own weight, mean that the number on the scale will move up at every weigh in! So although it is hard to do, accept that fact that you will see big changes and some weight gain this trimester. It is very necessary for the health of the mother and the baby. I was excited when my weight and measurements were "perfect"—right in the recommended range, and Dr. Heller said, "All your measurements are just perfect and the baby sounds great." It made me sure I was doing a great job for my baby and myself.

I needed that boost because this month there seemed to be more bad days than good days in the gym and on the track. My clients and boot camp recruits could see that I was showing a little bump and getting a bit slower, and I knew the day would come soon when I would be a lot slower and would be cheering them as they flew by me. I cannot even imagine how terrible I would have felt about myself had I not continued to exercise—what a blessing it was to be able to keep it up. I felt so slow and clumsy. But whenever I asked Steve how I looked, he wisely said, "You look beautiful!" I would smile and be glad for what I could still do in my workouts and racing. Despite my concerns, I always remembered that there is a difference between gaining weight and getting fat. I gained plenty of weight, but I was still pretty lean. Key thing to remember: *do not* work out to avoid weight gain. Make your training and racing be about your mental and emotional well-being and preparing for the event of your life! Don't try to avoid

"Kegels are the big joke to a lot of women. I thought, 'I'm fit—I'm don't need to run down the road doing Kegels.' But I learned my lesson the first time and did them while I ran the second time around. I found that if I did that motion, things stopped hurting. I wish I had done more Kegels early on. You think it's about not peeing on yourself, but really it's about your whole pelvic region."

—MOLLY, RUNNER, MOTHER OF TWO

gaining weight—relax and know that you will be able to lose it later. Just stay focused, enjoy the extra challenge, and get in some good workouts.

And go shopping! You may need to start looking at other workout clothes if your tighter-fitting tops or bottoms are getting a little *too* tight! You may need a bigger sports bra, too. Here are some more shopping tips:

- Look for clothes at inexpensive big box stores, such as Target. If you find clothes that work, stock up!
- For swimming, pick up a new regular racing suit one size larger (you don't need a maternity suit) and a swim cap to stay warm (your body will keep the baby warm first, so you may get cold in the water).
- Resist the urge to hide under XXL T-shirts. I tried that for awhile, but I learned that I felt better when I looked as good as I could.

- Schedule a shopping trip with a friend or a group of friends, to have more fun on the outing—especially if they are pregnant, too.

WORKING OUT

Over the next months, your center of gravity will move up and out, so starting now your fitness routines will accommodate and shift along with your increasing belly size. As your weight increases and the bump grows, your back, pelvis, hips, and legs will be stressed more in all your activities, not only your workouts. You may have some abdominal discomfort or low back pain as the ligaments that stabilize the pelvis, hips, and lower back stretch and loosen. If you get a backache, lift carefully. Keep moving and don't stand still too long. Above all, don't wear high heels! And don't mistake this for a sign that you should stop working out. These are simple signals to let you know that you need to make minor tweaks to your routine, whether it's different or modified exercises, more rest days between repeat workouts, or

---

TIP: STRENGTHEN YOUR PELVIC FLOOR

You've probably heard about Kegel exercises, especially as a remedy for incontinence. But Kegels actually strengthen the entire pelvic floor and do much more than just help you keep from peeing during your run.

Pregnancy and childbirth demand strong thigh, back, and abdominal muscles. Kegel exercises strengthen all the muscles of the pelvic floor, including the pubococcygeus muscle (PC muscle) you'll use to push the baby out. According to the Mayo Clinic, women with strong PC muscles feel more comfortable toward the end of their pregnancies when pressure increases in the pelvic floor.

To practice Kegels, tighten your muscles as if you're stopping urine and flatulence at the same time (check you've got the right muscles by stopping the flow of pee when you're on the toilet). Contract up and in; don't tighten your abs, hamstrings, or glutes. Here are two Kegel exercises:

Slow Kegels. These improve overall pelvic floor muscle strength. Breathe in. As you breathe out, slowly clench your pelvic muscles up as far as you can and hold for 5 seconds while breathing normally. Slowly release the muscles. Repeat 4 or 5 times, and gradually increasing the contraction time to 10 seconds.

Fast Kegels. Same as for Slow Kegels, but tighten and release your muscles quickly. Rest for at least 3 seconds between repetitions, and repeat up to 10 times.

a change in your diet to help with inflammation. But use your common sense—call your doctor if you experience any of the danger signs on page 5.

Common advice starting around now is to avoid supine exercises—moves done while lying flat on your back. In theory, the increased pressure of the uterus and placenta on your circulatory system can affect blood return to your heart. For this reason, swimmers should not spend a lot of time doing the backstroke, but continuing to spend some time doing the backstroke will help keep your posture tall as you work those back/posterior muscles. If you do begin to feel a bit lightheaded while on your back, you can always roll to your side. In general, you may continue with some supine activities as long as you keep moving; just don't lie still on your back for prolonged periods.

In Month 5 of my second pregnancy we traveled up to Lake Placid, New York, to watch the Ironman with a couple of friends, leaving Mackenzie (who just turned two) with my mother. When we arrived we all threw our wetsuits on and did one loop of the swim course for the Ironman. The water was amazing and swimming felt great. The next day we decided to go for a long bike ride on our Cross Bikes and set out for 40 to 50 miles on the Lake Placid course. I have to admit that I hated every minute of that ride. I felt slow and out of shape. The hills were brutal and I just kept thinking, "Why the F am I doing this?" I was miserable and yes, I could have been lying out in a lawn chair enjoying myself and my pregnancy, but that just wasn't me—and it's probably not you either. I actually enjoyed the challenge of not giving up and knowing that I could do it, even though it was pretty uncomfortable and I felt like I was sucking wind the entire time. When the ride was over I couldn't have been happier to get off that bike. But I felt great,

Expecting moms should be mindful of how much they use the Valsalva technique. The Valsalva technique, commonly employed in all kinds of lifting, is when the athlete takes a large inhale and fills the abdomen with air (creating internal stability) to assist with lifting a heavy load. This "hold your breath" technique is used during moves such as deadlifts and squats. However, repeated use of the Valsalva is not recommended in pregnant women. It can decrease oxygen consumption during activity (due to pressure on the thoracic vena cava) as well as potentially have negative impact on the athlete's pelvic floor and cause future incontinence issues.

Steve

knowing I overcame my negative thoughts and didn't talk myself out of doing it.

WHAT ABOUT GRAZING?

As an athlete, you may already be "grazing"—eating five or six smaller meals a day instead of three big chow-downs. This strategy is even more important when you are pregnant. Grazing helps regulate blood sugar. It helps you manage morning sickness by keeping a little food in your stomach. By the same token, it lessens heartburn because you never have a really full stomach.

Because they metabolize carbohydrates more quickly, pregnant women tend to become hypoglycemic faster, even if they never had problems with that before, especially if they don't have some protein and/or fat in the morning. Carbohydrates are digested quickly and, within an hour or two of eating, women can feel lightheaded or dizzy. Here are some healthy, low-glycemic-index snacks and mini meals that are easy to transport and enjoy postexercise, or really at any time. Because they are digested slowly, these low-glycemic-index foods or combinations won't spike your blood sugar.

> Deviled eggs with hummus
> Tuna with hummus
> Low-fat cottage cheese and fruit
> Tomatoes with cottage cheese
> Tomatoes and low-fat mozzarella cheese
> Veggies with dip
> Ham and fruit

"I went five or six months without missing a day of training, ever. Every day, I got up and went to the gym and I did *something*. I felt like if I went, even to just be around people, it was good to move and stay active. I loved it that, no matter what I did, everyone was so impressed. If I did one squat, everyone was saying 'Oh my god! Look at you!' It was awesome."

—HEATHER, CROSSFITTER, MOTHER OF THREE

You can also create an infinite variety of your own low-GI snacks/mini meals by choosing from the following options. Choose one protein, one carbohydrate, and one fat choice from the following lists.

Proteins

¼ cup low-fat cottage cheese

1 ounce part-skim or light mozzarella cheese

2 ounces part-skim or light ricotta cheese

1 ounce sliced turkey, ham, or chicken

1 ounce tuna packed in water

1 piece string cheese

1.5 ounce deli meat

Carbohydrates

½ apple

3 apricots

1 kiwi

1 tangerine

⅓ cup light fruit cocktail

½ pear

1 cup strawberries

¾ cup blackberries

½ orange

8 cherries

½ nectarine

1 peach

1 plum

½ cup crushed pineapple

1 cup raspberries

½ cup blueberries

½ grapefruit

Fats

3 green or black olives

1 macadamia nut

1 tablespoon avocado or guacamole

3 almonds

6 peanuts

2 pecans

½ teaspoon almond butter

½ teaspoon natural peanut butter

When should you eat? If you feel light-headed or if the baby is quieter after a long workout, these could be signs that you aren't eating enough or at the right times.

- Eat before working out to give you energy for the exertion.
- Eat during and immediately after long, hard workouts to make sure that enough food reaches the baby.
- Eat a snack 2 hours before bed so you don't fast for too long.

STAYING STRONG

This month's workout modifies familiar and intense activities to meet your needs. It's important to maintain upper and lower back strength, posture, and abdominal muscle tone. As your ligaments loosen, avoid back problems by working on posture: sit with your feet on a footstool; sleep with a pillow under your side; and use the strength in your legs, not your back, to lift heavy objects.

Once you begin to show, the baby has begun its move out of the protection of the pelvis. Because of this slight increase in vulnerability (mind you, the baby is still floating in the world's most amazing shock-absorber system!), some physicians may recommend you cut back on—or at least dial back the

---

THE PROS: LISA LESLIE, FOUR-TIME OLYMPIC GOLD-MEDAL BASKETBALL PLAYER

Lisa Leslie was one of the first players in the WNBA. After winning four gold medals, Lisa Leslie took a few years off from professional sports for the birth of her daughter. After the birth, instability in her hips made quick lateral movement more challenging, but her abs were stronger than ever. After she won her fourth gold in 2008, *Sports Illustrated* quoted her as saying, "My dream is to put on my four gold medals and run around the court with Lauren in my arms."

intensity of—ball sports (soccer, basketball, racquetball) or contact sports. If you are a rower, in theory there is risk of injury if the oar is caught in the water and the blade handle driven hard into the stomach (catching a crab), but the American Rowing Association reports no known incidents of such an injury to a pregnant woman.

Here's my weekly training plan for Month 5. Yours will reflect your own goals, as well as how you are feeling.

Sunday	Monday	Tuesday	Wednesday	Thursday	Friday	Saturday
Off or easy swim	Morning run, strength; evening bike	Morning boot camp run; evening swim	Morning bike, strength; evening short run	Morning track run; evening swim	Morning bike, strength	Morning strength, swim, bike, and/or run (a brick workout)

MONTH 5
STRENGTH WORKOUT

Suggested modifications: Focus on your posture now to keep your lower back strong. As your bump grows, your center of gravity will change—pay attention to balance!

If you do supine exercises, bend your knees for a neutral spine and keep the duration just long enough to finish your exercises. You should not lie motionless on your back, but as long as you keep moving (e.g., hollow body rock, dumbbell press, etc.) you will not compress the vena cava and impede the flow of blood from your lower body. Option: do exercises on your side, standing, or use a physioball to do more incline work so you are not lying flat. This month's workout includes an inverted—upside down—exercise. Inverted moves (handstand push-ups or modified handstand push-ups, for example) can be done at any stage of pregnancy if you are already experienced and comfortable with them. If you have never gone inverted, it is not recommended that you go inverted for the first time now! But if you have experience and feel comfortable doing so, go for it. Be mindful however of the length of time you spend upside down. As a result of vasodilation (wider blood vessels) you may feel a major rush of blood to your head and then, once righted, you may feel a bit dizzy. To help offset that, be sure to keep your core/midline tight and contracted as well as your legs. This will help with "venous return," or getting the blood back to the brain and heart.

Take note of any soreness in your pelvis or hips. Continue with your routine, but if you are more sore and uncomfortable than normal after a routine exercise, then your body is telling you to start modifying that movement. Be careful of your hips and lower back. Do not perform "developmental" stretches designed to increase or overextend the range of motion. Do not do hip adduction or abduction exercises. Don't overstress the quads; exercises that work the quads also stress the pelvic ligaments and can cause pain.

With the return of your energy, runners will want to get back on the track. Notice and adapt to your new center of gravity. Move to the treadmill for some workouts if you want.

As the center of gravity shifts, newer or more cautious cyclists might want to switch to a stationary bike in Month 5. As your belly grows, your knees and hips will have to splay outward to pedal around it. This could affect your ability to maintain your balance in unexpected situations. Limit off-road biking and, if you ride on the road, go with a buddy, carry your cell phone, and be sure to wear identification. You can always move to an indoor trainer or a spin class.

Novice weight lifters may want to move to the machines for more support and less danger to joints if ligaments feel loose. Alternatively, you can continue with your regular training practices but decrease the weight, speed of movement, and possibly your repetitions to help decrease the risk of injury.

Don't worry, you don't have to remember every modification. Just follow the workouts and listen to your body and its signals.

The Workout

Equipment needed: Agility ladder; medicine ball; dumbbells, barbell, pull-up bar

Dynamic Warm-up (see page 15)

Conditioning: "Fran": Complete the repetition sequence of 21, then 15, then 9 Barbell Thrusters and Pull-ups, moving from 21 thrusters to 21 pull-ups, 15 thrusters, 15 pull-ups, 9 thrusters, and finally 9 pull-ups as quickly as possible.

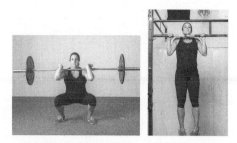

BARBELL THRUSTERS AND PULL-UPS

Strength Circuit (3 exercises): Complete this circuit 3 times

Exercise #1: Kettlebell Swings
  (Compound Movement)

Reps: 15

Exercise #2: Physioball Hamstring Curls
  (Pull focus)

Reps: 40

Exercise #3: Handstand/Pike Push-ups
  (Push focus)

Reps: 10

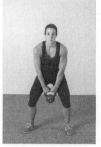

KETTLEBELL
SWINGS

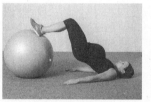

PHYSIOBALL
HAMSTRING CURLS

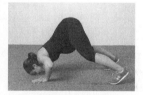

HANDSTAND/PIKE
PUSH-UPS

Cool Down and Stretch:
  Static stretch, mobility work, foam roller: Follow the Stretch Routine introduced on page 18.

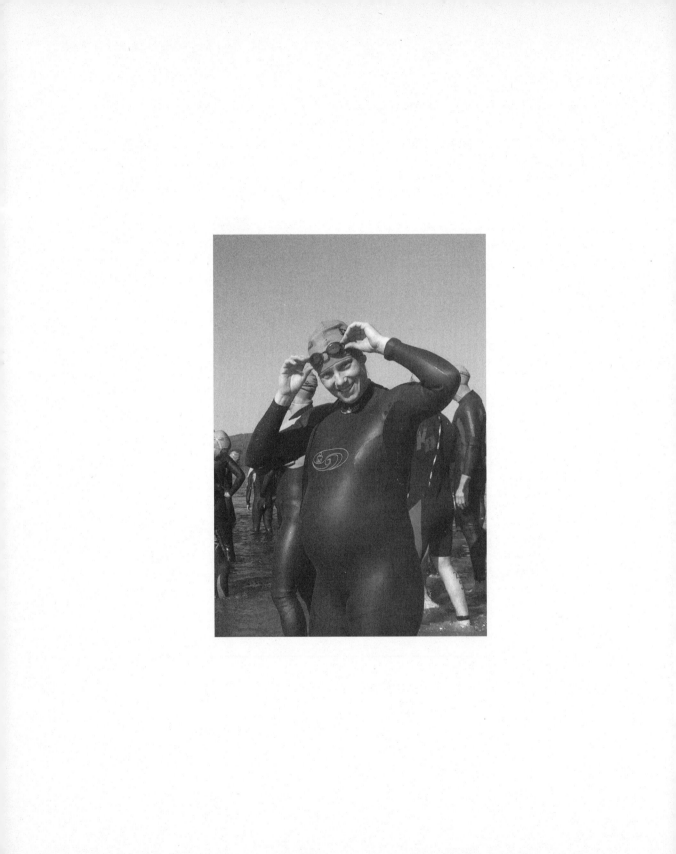

Not Giving Up My Jeans
(Thank You, Elastic Waistbands!)

Your Body Now

Strength	You are as strong as ever—keep it that way by being careful not to stress joints and ligaments that are loosened by hormones.
Agility	You may notice clumsiness, and your protruding belly will affect your balance.
Stamina	As the baby's position rises more, you may notice increased shortness of breath.
Well-being	Most women report that physically they feel great in the second trimester, despite pregnancy's side effects, but you may continue to have mood swings, irritability and forgetfulness. You may have a white vaginal discharge—caused by the same mechanism that brought you a runny nose, extra blood, and fluids in the mucous membranes. Like the runny nose, it will probably continue until delivery.
Nutrition	Your appetite is back with a vengeance!
Modifications	Avoid rapid side-to-side movements. If you feel faint while lying on your back, roll to your left side.
Your baby now	From head to toe, your baby is as long as an ear of corn (almost 12 inches) and weighs more than a pound; the baby kicks, pushes, and hiccups.

Have you noticed that you are getting clumsier and more forgetful with every passing month? It's not just a myth that pregnant women are likely to trip and drop things. A couple of things are going on in your body to support your nomination for Klutz of the Year. First, blame our old friend relaxin, which has loosened joints pretty much all over your body; the stretched ligaments and cartilage make your joints less stable (and more prone to injury), so be careful. But you're not going to turn into "Elastic Girl"; in fact, I noticed a big difference only when I went a little too heavy on the single-leg step-ups or squats. Swimming, biking, and running should not be affected by the relaxin. It's really a matter of paying attention to your environment and your body.

Another factor is "pregnancy brain." Yes, it's real! Many women report that it gets harder to concentrate as their pregnancy continues. Not paying attention can land you on your tush pretty quickly and get you some "looks" from your partner when you forget things!

DO YOU FEEL LIKE PUFF THE MAGIC DRAGON?

Another big contributor to clumsiness is all the fluid you are producing and retaining—50 percent more than normal, according to the American Pregnancy Association. These fluids are essential—they flush toxins from your system and the baby's—but they can cause your body to swell. If your hands swell, those puffy fingers are more likely to drop what they are holding and may make it more difficult to hold dumbbells, kettlebells, and barbells, so be mindful when using that equipment.

Fluid retention contributes to another one of those unexpected pregnancy side effects that may contribute to the dropsies: carpal tunnel syndrome. Extra fluids that accumulate in your hands all day compress the medial nerve and cause pain and tingling. It's often worse at night and early morning

OLD WIVES' TALE: IF YOU ARE CLUMSY DURING YOUR PREGNANCY YOU WILL HAVE A BOY.

Ha! If this were true, no girls would ever be born! Your weight has increased by 20 percent, your belly is sticking way out, and your center of gravity has shifted up and out. Your chances of being graceful are slim to none!

because the fluid distribution shifts. You may want to focus on exercises to strengthen your shoulders; this will help you to maintain better posture in the upper back and neck, which cause fluids to pool less and so may improve carpal tunnel symptoms. If you have wrist pain (especially during such exercises as bench dips, bear crawls, and crabwalks), elastic braces can help.

In fact, every part of you may seem to be expanding at this point—even your feet! You can thank relaxin for that, too—the looser ligaments let your feet spread out—and toss in some fluid retention, for good measure. Do you need new shoes? Go ahead and buy them—your feet will probably never return to their old size.

While you may never get your 7 narrows back, you can avoid or reduce the puffiness in the rest of your body by addressing the main causes of fluid retention:

- **Dehydration** causes the body to retain fluids. Drink more water and avoid hot, humid environments, especially

CHECKUP WITH DR. HELLER

Women often ask me about lying on their back and doing sit-ups or abdominal exercises while they are pregnant. Crunches are okay, but after eighteen to twenty weeks you should avoid lying flat on your back so that you don't cause circulatory issues. Between twenty and twenty-four weeks, the uterus grows above the bifurcation of the aorta and vena cava, just above the belly button. The vena cava is the main vein for returning blood to the heart, and the weight of the uterus can compress it if you are lying on your back (the supine position). You can still do crunches and other exercises, using a physioball because the ball will support you in an elevated position. Do this instead of lying flat on your back on a hard surface.

Ideally, by twenty-four weeks, you will be sleeping on your left side. Don't panic if you wake up on your back, and don't worry if you spend a moment or two on your back, especially if you are moving around. The fact is, if you are lying on your back and it is causing a problem, you will become aware of it and feel uncomfortable, lightheaded and short of breath. If pressure on the vena cava is slowing blood return, you will notice it; you will feel "off" and your natural inclination will be to change position. At that point, you just need to move or change position, and your circulation will take care of itself. Maintaining body awareness is the most important thing you can do during pregnancy; it will help you regulate your exercise regimen and make subtle changes in your daily life.

for your workouts. Cut back on diuretics, such as coffee and sodas.

- **Compromised circulation** from pressure of the uterus on the veins returning blood from the legs is improved by—you guessed it—exercise.
- **High salt intake** is addressed by taking a look at your diet. Avoid salty meals and snacks. Skip the junk food—it's loaded with sodium. Eat bananas, which are high in potassium; other natural diuretics are celery, onions, eggplant, garlic, parsley, and mint.

Best of all, find a time to put your feet up for a few minutes every day. Some women swear by swimming or even soaking in a cool tub. And remember to continue to drink plenty of water, no matter how bloated you feel! Keeping your urine light yellow in color will assure that you have enough fluids to flush your system. Your increased trips to the bathroom with make you want to avoid water, but you need to suck it up and drink to keep yourself healthy and on track. If you are tired of drinking plain water, try coconut water or snack on watery fruits and

---

TIP: MOSQUITO MAGNET

Is it just you, or are the mosquitoes really bad this year? It may be you! Mosquitoes put pregnant women high on their favorites list. Pregnant women exhale more carbon dioxide with every breath than other people do, and CO_2 is like catnip to mosquitoes. Also, your body temperature is slightly higher than other people's—another sure come-hither signal that will make mosquitoes choose you among all the people at the picnic. Fight back with a non DEET-based repellent and be sure to cover up after sundown.

---

vegetables such as cucumbers, watermelon, cabbage, iceberg lettuce, apples, bell peppers, pineapples, grapefruit, celery and berries. By consuming calorie-free liquids, eating healthy veggies and fruits, and monitoring your urine color, you can stay hydrated and feel good that you are getting plenty of nutrient-rich foods, too.

TAKING CARE OF THE BUMP

Another contributor to clumsiness is the baby bump. Your baby weighs a couple of pounds now, and the placenta and uterus itself are growing, too. Your uterus has risen above the pelvis, with the fundal height measuring about 25 cm, reaching just above your belly button. As you know from any lifting you have done, the closer the weight is to your core, the lighter it feels, and the farther away it is, the heavier it feels. As the baby's weight shifts away from your body's center, it "feels" heavier than its actual weight of only a few pounds. To add insult to injury, soon you won't be able to see your feet. Talk about clumsy!

Your wobbly joints, puffy fingers, and bigger belly combine to make your body behave very differently from what you are used to. As they feel more and more awkward, some women are concerned about falling and hurting the baby. As an expectant mom I worried about cycling until Dr. Heller reminded me that the baby is protected by the amniotic fluid, uterine membranes, and the abdominal muscles and bones. It's highly unusual for women who trip and fall—say, while dancing or running—to suffer adverse consequences in terms of contractions or a placental abruption. Most doctors tell women to avoid cycling during their pregnancy. Both my husband and my doctor supported my cycling during pregnancy, but I was very careful. My first pregnancy I did mostly spin classes at the gym through the winter; when the weather improved I got out on the road to prepare for the Season Opener triathlon in early May (two weeks before my due date). Steve went with me on all my outside rides; it made us both feel more secure in case of any difficulty. I purchased one of those super comfy gel seats—it was a godsend! During my second pregnancy, I felt very confident in my balance and stability so I was able to stick with my triathlon race bike through Month 8 with no issues except for my somewhat amusing form.

Just remember: If you are afraid of falling or have little confidence on the bike, you are more likely to fall. If you are confident in what you are doing and work within your comfort zone, you are less likely to take a fall. Do your best to stay within your limits, take the corners a bit easier, hit the brakes a bit sooner, get your shoes unclipped a bit earlier before coming to a stop, and choose routes that have less traffic.

I GET A KICK OUT OF YOU!

Some of the best moments of pregnancy are when you feel your baby move. By now, you are definitely feeling your baby's shifting around trying to get comfortable. You may even feel slight differences in the baby's apparent activity before and after your workouts. Some women notice less movement after they exercise, and this makes them worry that their activities are somehow harming the baby. A recent study of ultrasounds following exercise indicates that any changes in fetal movement, tone, or breathing after the mother's exercise tend to be slight and transient, and not a concern. In fact, at this point in the pregnancy, don't worry if you notice no movement for an afternoon or a day. Babies have sleep cycles, and respond to what you eat and drink, too. As you move through your day, you might even rock the baby to sleep.

"You have to be aware that your balance will be off. I was doing some ab exercises on the physioball at the gym, and the ball just popped out from under me. I was fine, of course, but the whole room gasped! Because my balance or footing could be off, I didn't run outside on any questionable roads or icy days."

—MOLLY, RUNNER, MOTHER OF TWO

Once you can distinguish the baby's moves from your own indigestion, you'll soon become familiar with your baby's normal pirouettes and schedule. Some medical teams encourage women to count movements during an active period each day (such as after a meal or moderate workout). Relax and note how long it takes the baby to move ten times. Keeping track of what's normal for your baby will help you notice activity changes if they occur.

It's pretty much a no-brainer that as the weight of the baby moves up and out, you will notice some strain in your back. You'll have more of a curve in your lumbar spine; this will tighten your lower back muscles. It didn't matter how fit I was, during both pregnancies I always felt that little strain in my lower back. Even though it was only a slight twinge during Month 6, it was there most evenings after a full day. Extra stretching of the lower back and hamstrings is definitely in order. And just think how much worse it would have been if you hadn't focused on your back and core in the early months!

Back pain is probably the most common muscular complaint from pregnant women. During pregnancy, the hip flexors and piriformis shorten as the pelvis tilts forward. Strengthening the hip extensors (the back of the thighs) and stretching the hip flexors will help address lower back pain. Planks are great for strengthening your core. If you use the machines at your gym, strengthen your quads and hamstrings with the leg extension and leg curl machines. Work your lats to help keep your posture upright.

Pay attention to your form when working your core. Don't "crank" your neck when you do crunches. Instead, draw in the abdomen to press your belly button against your spine. In fact, instead of doing a lot of crunches, stick with planks (front and side)—those exercises alone will keep your core strong. Just holding planks can get very boring, so add other core exercises that force you to hold the plank position while moving arms, legs or both, and add weight/resistance for variety.

If you do have back pain, consider where it's coming from and when it started. Is this a problem you had before you were pregnant, or did it start after you got pregnant and, if so, when during your pregnancy did the pain start? If this is a chronic problem, pregnancy may exacerbate it, especially in the third trimester as the added weight in the front of the body pulls everything forward. Incorporating more stretching exercises for the front of the body (quad and hip flexors) and then strengthening the posterior (back of the body) muscles will help. Strengthen the lower back, hamstrings, glutes, mid- and upper back—all of which will help you feel better and decrease the discomfort. Be mindful of how long you are sitting as well—especially if you do not sit correctly—and be sure your chair supports your back. As most of us sit forward on our chair to do desk work, this leaves our lower back unsupported, overstretching our glutes and shortening our hip flexors. This increases tightness in the front and weakness in the back. Just a few minor changes can be helpful to decrease or even eliminate back pain and discomfort.

A helpful solution for back pain, pulled from the physical therapy world, is to use an elastic support belt. Brandi used one during the 5-mile road race she ran a few days before the delivery of our son, Maddox. But many women wear these belts much earlier in pregnancy to help the lower back manage the load. It can be worn during exercise and training bouts, or wear it at work or around the house if you don't like the compression sensation for workouts. Most people who are prone to or suffering from back problems enjoy the support these belts provide, and it is a cost-effective way to relieve the physical strain from your posterior chain (hamstrings, glutes, lower, mid-, and upper back).

Steve

EATING FOR TWO—AT LAST!

Morning sickness is a distant memory and you have a healthy appetite now! Be sure you are eating enough to fuel your baby's growth and your own activities without putting on unnecessary pounds. In fact, you can start adding a couple hundred extra calories about now, above and beyond the amounts that compensate for your workouts. Get your nutrients but leave the empty calories on the grocery store shelves. Buy nonfat milk and yogurt and save ice cream for an occasional treat. Indulge in plenty of raw fruits and vegetables (take a pass on broccoli if it gives you heartburn!). Not only do fruits and crudités fill you up "for free," calorically speaking, but they are also packed with fluids and fiber (both of which help with constipation and hemorrhoids). Remember to graze: five or six small meals will keep your blood sugar and energy levels where they need to be, and will reduce heartburn.

WORKING OUT IN MONTH 6

Like many women, I had some pelvic pain at around the six-month mark. If you do, stop the longer distance running and stick with shorter, high-intensity running and plyometrics for your cardio workout. Consider switching from running to a spin class if the abdominal pressure gets uncomfortable.

But during my second pregnancy I could run through the whole nine months and for the most part I felt great and hit some good paces. One day I even challenged my recruits to keep up with me on stair repeats! This was very empowering and made me feel amazing. I felt strong in every way. The good days like this are few and far between at this point, so when you have one, cherish the moment and be sure to brag about it!

> "My ob-gyn was totally behind me. I asked her, 'Is there a point when I should stop working out?' She said, 'At thirty-six weeks you might want to stop running. You'll be carrying a lot of weight then.' I did whatever I wanted as long as it felt OK."
>
> —PAULA, RUNNER, MOTHER OF TWO

Then I had the other days. You'll have them too, the days that challenge you physically, mentally, and emotionally—the days when you work so damn hard to go so damn slow. You might get cramps and have to walk mid set, or feel clumsy and slow and get down on yourself. But keep chugging along the best you can and remind yourself, "It's worth it, so do it."

Even if you are able to keep at it, by the sixth month running is more difficult and can be very uncomfortable at times. After all, you have a definite bump, and your pelvic ligaments may not appreciate all that bouncing around. If you do keep running, you need to ask yourself: "How much discomfort can I tolerate to get in a run or track workout, knowing that will help me more mentally and

PAULA RADCLIFFE, WORLD RECORD MARATHONER

A champion in the marathon, half marathon, and cross-country, Paula Radcliffe left at the top of her career in the 2006 season because she was expecting her first child. She dropped from competition, but she did not stop training. On the contrary, she trained harder than most nonpregnant women—running 140 miles a week and not skimping on the hill repeats. In her seventh month, she replaced one of her two daily runs with a stationary bike ride. She returned to training twelve days after giving birth, saying, "I felt a bit wobbly, but I was glad to have my body back." Radcliffe made her marathon return at the 2007 New York City Marathon, which she won with an official time of 2:23:09.

Radcliffe told *The Telegraph*, "I've read that if you exercise when you are pregnant, your babies turn out more intelligent, do well on their Apgar tests and handle the distress of labor better," she says. "Besides, if I couldn't run for nine months, I'd go insane. When I run, I sort out my problems."

emotionally than it will physically?" Remember, it is easy to stop and walk when you need to and you can modify your run distance and intensity accordingly. If you do run and you feel pressure or strain in your belly, buy yourself a belly band. It will support your belly and help control the bouncing. You can even use a lifting belt, which you can purchase at a hardware store. While you are at it, buy yourself some compression socks. As your pregnancy continues, your feet and ankles might swell, and the socks will help with return blood flow. Increasing the time you take to cool down as well as icing after workouts may also be helpful. Icing your lower extremities will not only reduce muscle damage as a result of the exercise bout, but it will also help with any swelling due to hormonal influences and water retention.

I was able to continue track workouts with my training group until the end of my seventh month. After that, I dropped track and long endurance runs and only jogged short distances (3–4 miles) mixed with strength work such as Burpees (jumping only as high as I felt comfortable), push-ups (depending on the size of my bump, of course!) squats, and abs. From now on, the workouts in this book reflect these changes: they are still challenging, but with less running and modified metabolic routines. But if you are feeling good and getting in those long runs, keep at it!

Whatever you have to do to accommodate your condition, don't stop your workouts. You have made it this far, so there is no excuse now unless the doctor says otherwise. Stopping exercise late in pregnancy has very unfortunate outcomes for the baby's size and

"You just modify the exercises as you go along—it's fun to get creative about it. Instead of Supermans, do Superdogs. Use the stability balls more at an incline for balance. Sit on a bench for V-ups instead of than lying on your back doing the suitcases. Squats instead of squat jumps because it felt a little better to me to not be jumping. That kind of thing."

—SUSAN, BOOT CAMP ATHLETE, MOTHER OF ONE

mother's overall weight gain. According to a study by Dr. James F. Clapp, women who exercised strenuously for the early months but stopped in late pregnancy have the biggest babies of all—bigger and fatter, with almost 3 percent more body fat. You may remember that exercise in early pregnancy stimulates the placenta's growth and efficiency, making your body and your baby better prepared for emergencies. Women who stop exercising late in pregnancy effectively hand over their calories to that highly efficient placenta to give to the baby. The result is a fatter baby. I for one did not want a fat baby, especially given the epidemic of overweight children today. Not to mention my slightly selfish desire to make delivery as easy as possible, so far as it was in my control! So I kept at it, following a schedule like this one.

Sunday	Monday	Tuesday	Wednesday	Thursday	Friday	Saturday
Off or easy swim	Morning run, strength; evening bike	Morning boot camp run; evening swim	Morning bike, strength; evening short run if I feel up to it	Morning track run; evening swim	Morning bike, strength	Morning strength, swim, bike, and/or run (a brick workout)

SAMPLE MONTH 6
STRENGTH WORKOUT

Suggested modifications: Be sure to support your abdomen and breasts if you are still running long distances. If running is too uncomfortable or at all painful, find an alternate cardio activity—the elliptical or rowing machines, swimming, or stationary bike. If your belly interferes with push-ups or burpees, do incline push-ups instead and squat thrusts instead.

Continue to assess and discontinue or modify any activity that makes you feel shaky or off balance. By now you have given up downhill skiing, skating, horseback riding, off-road biking, and trail running. Good replacements are swimming, stationary bike (recumbent might be more comfortable), rowing machine, treadmill. If you are cycling or running outside, stay away from high-traffic areas. If you still enjoy step aerobics, use a low step if you aren't confident in your balance. If yoga is your sport, cut out back bends, lying still on your stomach or back, and inverted poses. Cyclists, put away the racing bike for one with wider tires and a carriage that lets you sit more upright. Adjust your seat and handlebar height. Clipless pedals will make the mount and dismount feel more stable.

For swimmers, the breaststroke strengthens the chest muscles and shortens the back muscle, promoting good alignment. For a nice rest, use a snorkel with breaststroke arms and crawl legs—it gives your back a rest from popping your head out of the water.

If you are playing tennis, keep your pace moderate. Play doubles and let the other player pick up the slack. Rapid lateral motion is tricky, so pay attention to your balance.

The Workout

Equipment needed: Dumbbell, medicine ball; tubing; pull-up bar; tire

Dynamic Warm-up (see page 15)

Conditioning: 20-yard sprints/accelerations with 10-second rest times 6

Strength Circuit (4 exercises): Complete this circuit 3 times

Exercise #1: Overhead Squat > Broad Jump (Compound and Plyometric)

Reps: 10 squats immediately into 10 broad jumps—no rest between exercises

Exercise #2: Dumbbell Push-Press > Dynamic Push-up (Compound Movement and Push focus)

Reps: 10 push-presses immediately into 5 push-ups—no rest between exercises

Exercise #3: Side Bridge hold (Core focus)

Reps: 30 seconds per side

Exercise #4: Ring/TRX Row > Bent Over, Straight-arm Tubing Pullbacks (Pull focus)

Reps: 10 per side immediately into 20 pullbacks—no rest between exercises

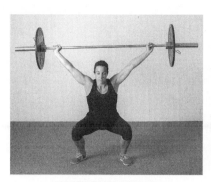

OVERHEAD SQUAT

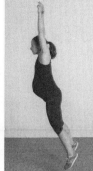

BROAD JUMP

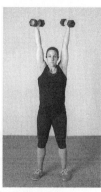

DUMBBELL
PUSH-PRESS

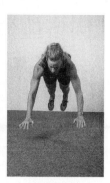

DYNAMIC
PUSH-UP

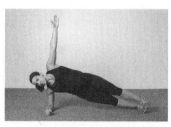

SIDE BRIDGE HOLD

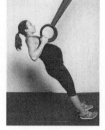

RING/TRX ROW

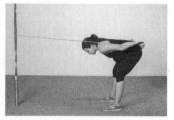

BENT OVER, STRAIGHT-ARM
TUBING PULLBACKS

Conditioning: Sledgehammer Tire Slam
Tabata (No tire or sledgehammer?
Substitute Medicine Ball Wood Chops
Tabata)

    4 minutes: Hit tire 20 seconds, rest 10
    seconds. Repeat for 8 rounds.

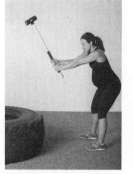

SLEDGEHAMMER
TIRE SLAM

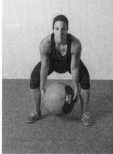

MEDICINE BALL
WOOD CHOPS

Cool Down and Stretch:

    Static stretch, mobility work, foam roller: Follow the Stretch Routine introduced on page 18.

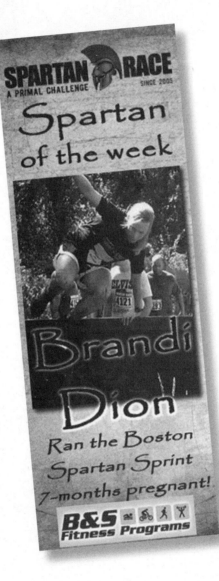

Running Through Molasses, but Still Running!

Your Body Now

Strength	Your muscles are as strong as ever, but loose pelvic ligaments can limit lifting.
Agility	Agility? What's that?
Stamina	You may feel winded during and after exertion as the baby's position rises into your rib cage.
Well-being	Many women experience a burst of energy in the third trimester, along with some excitement. Did I mention increased forgetfulness?
Nutrition	Continue to take in about 300 extra "high-quality" calories per day.
Modifications	Curtail single-leg work; be cautious in or curtail any high-impact activity, such as jumping.
Your baby now	As big as a coconut, more than 16 inches long and weighing more 3½ pounds, the baby can hear your voice and heartbeat.

Welcome to the third trimester! You are definitely feeling and looking pregnant! If you haven't looped that hair elastic through the buttonhole of your jeans to give you a few more weeks as I did, your old jeans are hanging in the closet and you've moved on to clothes that accommodate the "bump." After all, the baby is about 15 to 16 inches long now and might weigh as much as 4 pounds; with the placenta and extra fluids, you've probably added 15 pounds and are putting on more at the rate of about a pound a week. Maybe if you throw on a baggy sweatshirt you can still pull off the "no show," but most of the time there's no way you can carry that around without everyone wondering, not "if" but "when?"

This was one of the toughest times for me, especially in my first pregnancy when it was all new. Sometimes I was just uncomfortable no matter what I wore! My gym shorts felt awkward with the waistband below the belly and that unaccustomed tightness in the butt. One day I stepped on the treadmill to warm up before hitting the weights and got so irritated with feeling bad in my clothes, running with a big belly that felt tight and in the way, and being winded after five minutes of jogging that I slammed the big red Stop button on the treadmill and stomped over to Steve with an attitude. He saw me coming and tried to look away but I didn't let him escape. I started complaining about *everything* I was going through and, like the good partner he is, he just listened and listened and listened. I am sure he was thinking, "What the hell do I say and not get my head ripped off?!" but I was genuinely in need of an emotional boost and counted on him to provide one. So Steve looked at me nearly in tears, gave me a big hug and said "You look so beautiful and I am so proud of you for even coming here and sticking to your routine. Get through what you can and we'll leave when you are ready." Then he gave me a kiss and told me to go back to working out. I was still pretty miserable but his kiss and telling me I was

---

OLD WIVES' TALE: EXERCISE CAN CAUSE PREMATURE DELIVERY OR LOW BIRTH WEIGHT.

This idea can be traced back to research that shows that some kinds of on-the-job work stress are associated with early delivery. But the work stresses in question involve long periods of standing in one position, protracted walking, or heavy lifting. The culprits are most likely dehydration and blood pooling in the legs (the pregnancy-relaxed leg veins have a harder time pumping it back to the heart), leading to fatigue and low blood pressure. Exercise has the opposite effects.

In fact, Dr. James Clapp's studies show that while continuing regular and vigorous exercise through pregnancy does not increase the incidence of preterm membrane rupture or labor, more regular exercisers do deliver in Weeks 38 and 39 (not prematurely, but before their due dates). More nonexercisers deliver in Weeks 40, 41, and 42.

---

beautiful gave me the boost and motivation that I needed to get through that particular night at the gym. Thank goodness I only experienced a few of those extreme moments of misery and self-doubt during my workouts and pregnancies. But all the ingredients are there—your hormones are raging and your body has changed almost beyond recognition. If your partner doesn't happen to be there for your meltdown, let me tell you:

CHECKUP WITH DR. HELLER

We have to realize that yes, there are certain risks to any athletic activity, but Mother Nature has provided for most natural events. Statistically the risk of injury is much higher just getting behind the wheel of a car. The most common serious injuries to the mother and potentially the baby involve automobile accidents or falls on stairs. But when you participate in such activities as biking and skiing, you can't control the behavior and risk-taking of others. That's why I recommend that women avoid these sports late in the pregnancy except in rare and managed circumstances—you never know when another person is going to do something that will put you in danger, and you will be less able to do the fancy footwork necessary to avoid an accident.

You are fabulous for showing up and doing your workouts. Do what you can. Show up again tomorrow.

NO DOUBT ABOUT IT, YOU LOOK PREGNANT!

And how do you feel? Some women feel just great. They even get a big burst of energy in the third trimester. There are a couple of reasons for this. If you suffered a lot from morning sickness, then you know how great it is to enjoy eating again! Your body will put those calories to good use, and you'll have more energy that you did when you were chewing on soda crackers and ice cubes. Some women just "hit their stride" around Month 7 and start nesting and preparing for the baby. On the other hand, some women start to feel a bit run down at this time. In addition to eating for two, they are running, climbing stairs, and in fact doing *everything* for two! Or they

may have trouble sleeping now that they are getting bigger—immobility, leg cramps, or bladder pressure can make for wakeful nights and affect your performance during the day. And with the uterus crowding your other organs, don't be surprised if you still have heartburn or indigestion. Starting early in the third trimester, I had really bothersome nighttime heartburn until I learned to eat smaller meals and to wait at least two or three hours between supper and bedtime. Elevating the head of my mattress helped; sleeping on my side, propped up with pillows, also improved my sleep, but I still woke up at night with fish burps and heartburn! All I thought was "When will this be over?" and I still had about two months to go.

At least now there is no possibility of confusing your own heartburn for the baby's movements. You should continue to be aware of your baby's normal patterns. Contact your midwife or doctor if:

- You don't feel ten or more separate movements while lying on your side for two hours.
- Your baby doesn't start to move in response to noise or some other stimulus.
- There's a big decrease in your baby's movements, or a gradual decrease over several days.

But most likely your baby is just taking a snooze for a while, and will keep you awake with kicks and flips as soon as you turn out the light. If you feel lightheaded, or if the baby seems extra quiet after a long workout, you may not be eating enough or at the right times. Make sure that both you and the baby get enough food by fueling during and immediately after you exercise. Trust me, by the end of this month your definition of a "long, hard workout" will have changed! But if you are trying to keep a good run or cycling base during pregnancy, proper fueling will be important. Remember—if you are working out you are burning calories so be sure to compensate for those calories with extra healthy snacks. And remember that gaining

One of my fondest memories of Brandi's pregnancies was doing the Spartan Race together. (See Brandi's recap of the same race on page 117.) We made a little sign for her belly that said "CAUTION: 7 Months Pregnant" and I had such a blast watching her taking it to the race. In all honesty, I was looking forward to the obstacles because the pace she was keeping was getting me winded. If you watch the video you can hear me panting in the back! But you can also hear my exuberance and pride when I tell the volunteer soldiers that my seven-months pregnant wife was beating all these other "Spartans." Watching her take the last incline wall obstacle with ease gave me this great sense of awe: my wife can do anything and she kicks ass. Brandi ended up being the first Spartan they highlighted when they created the Spartan Blog.

Cheering at competitions and events is only one way to support your pregnant athlete partner. By now she (or rather, the baby) is really showing, and your workouts at the gym, on the streets, or on the trail may be getting some odd looks from people around you. Just keep reassuring her that she looks great and she is doing the right thing for her and the baby. Other little things you can do for her during these weeks and months include keeping track of her exertion rate via the "talk test" when you are working out and creating intentional breaks by starting a conversation if she begins to show signs of overdoing it. However, if she doesn't want any distractions and wants to work out uninterrupted, giving moral support or helping set up the weights may be all she needs. Just being there with her is what makes the experience meaningful. Put yourself in her place and remind her how special she is to you and how proud you are of her.

Steve

weight changes your basal metabolic rate, so add calories to support the weight you have gained.

Because your baby is growing so fast, eat 300 calories a day just for the baby and make every calorie count. In the third trimester I was even more careful about eating foods rich in the nutrients vital to my health and the baby's. I chose foods from all the different food groups at every meal and snacked "generously." If you expect to gain the full 25 to 40 pounds recommended by the College of Gynecologists and Obstetricians, you can enjoy quite a nice variety of good food and treats to support your workouts. And women who exercise through their pregnancies gain an average of 8 pounds less than those who don't—it's okay to gain a *normal* but *below average* amount. So eat wisely, but don't skimp! Don't be afraid to gain the proper amount of weight. A varied and healthy diet is beneficial in more ways than one: recent research indicates that your baby can actually *taste* what you are eating! And babies that taste carrots and spinach now are more likely to eat them when they have a choice. Not sure I believe this—my kids aren't exactly begging for green beans or Brussels sprouts, but they do love broccoli and if this idea helps you eat healthier, then it is worth trying.

PRACTICE CONTRACTIONS

After the sixth month, you will start to have Braxton Hicks contractions that become more frequent as the weeks go by. These harmless "practice" contractions are some-times so strong that they can trigger false labor and send you on a trip to the hospital. Exercise stimulates uterine activity, so an active woman will experience progressively more cramps during late-pregnancy exercise. Those cramps usually stop shortly after the end of the workout; if they persist for more than 20 or 30 minutes after your workout, true labor may not be far off. I did experience a few uncomfortable cramps during some boot camp and track workouts. Each time they hit, I would slow down, put my hand under the belly and think, "Am I *crazy* to be out here doing this?" The cramps would go away and I would resume my run! The cramps gave me a good excuse to slow down and spend some extra time with my slower recruits or track runners. I never told them I was having cramps—that was my little secret as I worked through it. Remember that Braxton Hicks contractions should stop after a half hour or so; if the contractions don't stop, then they may be signaling the real thing!

BIGGER AND BETTER

Your belly is expanding and you can expect it to bump into things as you try to squeeze through spaces that were never a problem until you were *this* pregnant—before you had a bump that feels as big as a basketball sticking out in front. At some point late in the first or early in the second trimester you will completely discontinue prone (face-down) floor exercises—you don't need me to tell you that lying on your stomach can be extremely uncomfortable!

On the plus side (sort of!), your breasts continue to get bigger—a great perk of pregnancy for us smaller-breasted women! Unfortunately, if you are a runner or do a lot of plyometrics/jumping or high-impact aerobics, all the bouncing of your breasts and belly can be uncomfortable. And your breasts may even have started leaking a few drops of colostrum now and then. You may want to invest in some larger sport bras; if one doesn't give enough support, try wearing two, and tuck in some nursing pads if you are leaking. Once you get the bouncing under control (or just get used to the feeling) you can continue any cardio or endurance training in the third trimester, as long as you don't push to exhaustion. Listen for your body to tell you when you need to slow down or stop. Keep your perceived exertion at the "somewhat hard" level.

Loosened joints and weight redistribution will add to your overall clumsy feeling, making speed, acceleration, and sudden lateral motion seem like distant memories. You may feel that you will never get them back. But trust me you will, and sooner than you think. But for now, you have started to recognize that there are some moves you shouldn't be making. No one likes to fall—it hurts and it's embarrassing! The main injury will probably be to your pride; the baby is nestled in those membranes, abdominal muscles, and fluids. But a twisted ankle or sprained wrist could put you out of commission for a month, so be cautious and pay attention. This goes double if you are still doing agility work or running on uneven terrain.

> "I gained almost 40 pounds, but I wasn't really worried about it. I knew it would come it off quickly once I got back on the water."
>
> —SARAH, ROWER, MOTHER OF TWO

Surprisingly, some exercises may actually become easier as your pregnancy progresses. The increased amount of blood in your circulatory system now reverses the conditions of low blood volume that may have made you dizzy and nauseous during the first few months. With more blood in the system, your heart pumps a greater volume of blood with each beat, sending more oxygen to your muscles and the baby. Some women notice that their heart rates don't climb very high in the third trimester no matter what they do. Throughout my pregnancies I never felt that I had to make a conscious effort to go easy—my body just made it impossible to go real hard. By this I mean that my RPE on a 9-minute-mile run in the last trimester was the same as it was at a 7-minute-mile pace during the first trimester. Even though I was working just as hard, my body could not go at the old speed. Simply put, I was working really hard to go very slow! The tricks your heart rate can play in the third trimester are another reason to rely on perceived exertion to gauge the intensity of your workouts. Don't ever feel bad about your pace or performance—that's the last thing you should worry about. Just be thankful, as I was, to be able to work out and even race up until the day you give birth. Improved oxygen management means that some women can slightly *exceed* their prepregnancy performance; at the very least it increases your tolerance to heat stress.

MAKE THAT *DRINKING* FOR TWO!

It's especially important to stay cool, hydrated, rested, and well fed. If you are exercising, then your body is hot, and hydrating helps you maintain your body temperature at levels that don't stress the baby. Water cleans waste—yours and the baby's—from your system.

Remember that your blood volume has doubled so you have to drink a lot to maintain your hydration and salt intake. Have a big drink first thing in the morning and when you get up during the night. Drink during every workout. Keep track of your water intake—eight 8-ounce servings is the minimum! Keep the calories low by making cool water your drink of choice. Your urine should be pale yellow. Avoid exercising in hot and humid conditions: no lunchtime runs, hot gyms, hot tubs, sauna, or steam baths.

DON'T BE AFRAID TO KEEP PUSHING YOURSELF

For both my pregnancies, little things bugged me (like the heartburn at night!), my big belly, my slower pace, but truthfully I had little to complain about. As pregnancies go, I had it pretty easy. I didn't really change my workout intensity level because my body controlled what I could do and how hard I could push it by just slowing down naturally. And I really enjoyed the challenge of seeing what I could accomplish as my due dates got closer. Everyone asked, "How long will you be working out? Are you going to keep biking? When are you going to stop lifting?" Those questions baffled me. I wondered, "Why are they asking me that? Why would I stop?" And why should I? I had no pain; I wasn't forcing anything. I was just doing what I always did: working out every day and doing what I was accustomed to. I wasn't doing this to avoid

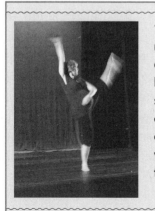

"As a dancer, I had continued to dance and teach through pregnancy. I had the idea that I wanted to perform at the recital—the end of my seventh month—but only really decided a day or so before. When I told the lighting designer, 'Surprise! I've added a solo!' he was shocked. 'Really?! Are you joking?' The entire tech crew thought it was a joke. Afterward, they were amazed. And during the concert, the audience was great. Afterward, one older woman came up to me and just held my hand for a long time. I felt empowered and so strong."

—MEGHAN, DANCER, MOTHER OF ONE

gaining weight, I did it because I loved it and it was my life. It was a part of me. Besides, I knew that it would help me through labor and delivery and speed my recovery.

Other athletes feel the same way—in fact, they take it a step beyond me. Carol worked out until the day before she delivered. Heather taught a double spin class and a boot camp class the morning of the delivery of her second child. You may hang up your sneakers at Month 7, or you may run the Chicago Marathon on your due date, as Amber Miller did. My point is to listen to your body and do the best you can. No more and no less.

So even though there's a lot going on physically, mentally, and emotionally with you and your body, and you feel very big, awkward, and uncomfortable, don't be afraid to keep pushing yourself especially through your bad days and moments. By that I mean going that extra distance before you need to stop, and doing as much as you can do—here's the key word: safely. I always challenged myself to keep doing what I do as long as I could. Look to your partner and friends to pick you up when you need it.

It's also helpful to think ahead and create goals for yourself. Registering for a friendly race or other competition can be a great way to keep your mind off the discomforts and miseries of pregnancy, even if you decide against competing come race day. Challenge yourself to see how well you can do! It's even okay to compete, even if it's just to catch that person in front of you. Just keep it up—remember, you can do this and you need this! If you made it through the entire second trimester exercis-

ing regularly, then you can make it through the last trimester. Whether it's strength training, boot camp, running, swimming, cycling, or body-weight activities, at any volume of 30-plus minutes, anything you do will be a big benefit to you and the baby. But remember, it's okay to step back, too, if you need to. You've been taking great care of yourself and your baby; some days you just may not feel like working out—and that's okay.

If you do sign up for a race, you aren't running to win, of course, and your friends and family may be a little taken aback by your plans ("Huh? You are going to do what?"). But if you are working out and feel strong, you can take it as a mental challenge and even have fun with it, as I did.

KEEP YOUR MEDICAL TEAM ON BOARD

Luckily, Dr. Heller continued to be encouraging and supportive through all my adventures. Doctors' appointments are always exciting when you're pregnant, and the third trimester is extra special. I loved listening to the heartbeat. During these months of training and racing, every checkup had the same report: my belly and baby measured perfectly. Things could not have been better. Things were going so well that it almost seemed that the doctor and I talked more about racing and working out than about the baby. That's one of the things I love about him: he is an athlete who loves hearing about my workouts and racing and telling us his stories. When my nonathletic friends heard

THE SPARTAN RACE

At the start of Month 7 of my second pregnancy, I was registered for a Spartan Race, a 5K with military-style obstacles including 4- and 8-foot walls, a slanted rope wall, barbed wire crawl, mud pit, cargo nets, water hoses, fire pit, and Spartan Jousters waiting at the end, for good measure.

This race was an "OMG" experience. How would I get over those walls? My belly seemed huge and was bound to get in the way. The fire pit and barbed wire crawl sounded pretty sketchy. But I was confident in my physical abilities and—this was key—I never felt that I would be putting my little "traveling companion" in danger. I was prepared to take my time and be careful. If I didn't feel safe or able to complete an obstacle I would just do the push-ups or whatever alternative punishment they allowed people to do in order to move on. And Steve would be racing alongside me to be sure that all was well along the course and help me if needed. In short, I approached the event less as a contender than as a very pregnant lady. If I couldn't run, I'd walk. I had no expectations; I just wanted to have fun. And that I did!

So when the starting gun went off, so did I! I charged the very steep and long first hill (by "charge" I mean "sucking wind to make it to the top") and kept going, feeling good. I walked only when I had to—when there were slow people in front of me ("Out of my way! Prego coming through!" ha-ha) or at lines at obstacles. I made it over and through every obstacle, needing help only at the 6-foot-high rope wall, where my belly kept getting caught on the top rope. Steve gave me a lift so I could do a body flip over the rope wall. To my surprise (and to the astonishment of onlookers) I landed on my feet—now *that* was scary for a second, exciting for the next second, and funny as we jogged on! If you are seven months pregnant and looking for a little inspiration—or good laugh—check out the video (http://www.bnssport science.com/pregnancy-training/)—it is a sight to see!

Besides actually clearing the wall, what most surprised me that day was how good I felt. I had had some tough running workouts that challenged me mentally so I was prepared for the worst. Instead I enjoyed the amazing feeling of crossing that finish line. Besides, it was fun to see people's shocked expressions as they noticed I was pregnant, and seven months pregnant at that!

how supportive and encouraging he was of my fitness goals, they could hardly believe he was a real doctor! I just laughed; he was a great supporter of my somewhat extreme workout habits and of his other active pregnant clients as well.

WORKING OUT

Other challenges motivated me. How long could I keep up with the workouts in my conditioning class? How long could I keep leading my boot camp clients through their

6:00 to 7:00 a.m. routine? I was still able to bike, cautiously, although my legs were starting to veer to the outside of my belly as I pedaled, so this was "interesting" to say the least! The most dramatic changes in my workouts involved single-leg exercises. I felt strong in my first pregnancy (and didn't have a book like this one to guide me), but at some point I should have lightened up on my weight load rather than thinking I should be able to squat the same as before. I didn't lighten up, and this resulted in some pelvic imbalances that then led to some minor pelvic soreness. With the loosening of the ligaments in my hips, the single-leg plyometrics and dynamic movements had to become more static, and the static single-leg exercises had to be taken to two feet.

You don't have to stop or even cut back on your program, just be smart with the weight load. You can still get in a great workout if you make a few modifications. This month's workouts will help you maintain intensity without losing your balance or stressing joints and ligaments, even as that bump gets bigger. Up until now we've been doing a lot of exercises standing on one leg to build core strength and balance, but from now on the single-leg rows and presses are off the list. Instead, plant both feet on ground and focus on form.

You can continue other floor exercises, stretching, and weight training for short periods. Don't lie motionless on your back to rest between sets—ACOG advises that you avoid lying still on your back (supine position) as that position can cause "relative obstruction of venous return and, therefore, decreased cardiac output and orthostatic hypotension" (in other words, lightheadedness). But blood flow should not be a problem if your legs and torso are moving. My experience bears this out: I never had this sensation when doing floor exercises, such as abs, floor press, and so forth but I did feel lightheaded during an ultrasound! Use common sense: if you continue doing any floor exercises on your back, stop and roll onto your left side if you feel dizzy.

This month's workouts help you maintain intensity without losing your balance or stressing your joints and ligaments, even as that bump gets bigger. Keep to your schedule as well as you can.

Sunday	Monday	Tuesday	Wednesday	Thursday	Friday	Saturday
Off	Morning run, strength; evening bike	Morning run; evening swim	Morning bike, strength; evening short run if feeling up to it	Morning track run; evening swim	Morning bike, strength	Morning strength, swim, bike, and/or run (a brick workout)

MY MONTH 7 STRENGTH WORKOUT

Suggested modifications: Your center of gravity has shifted, and acceleration and sudden lateral shifts are more difficult. As your ligaments loosen, pay attention to your body and curtail single-leg work. Go easy on squats if your pelvis is sore the next day.

If you are a cyclist, use caution if you are riding outside. A recumbent bike may be more comfortable, putting less pressure on your bladder, bowel, lungs, and other organs.

If you are a rower, you'll find you need to let the belly bump go between your knees on the catch; this will weaken your leg drive somewhat.

If you are running, a body gel/paste will help reduce chafing. For most triathletes or long-distance runners, Vaseline or BodyGlide are essentials to prevent chafing. Spreading these products to other parts of the body is not such a bad idea, especially if you begin to feel chafing in spots where you are not accustomed to it.

Start to cut back on any jumping—aerobics, box jumps, jump rope—in the last months.

The Workout

Equipment needed: Kettlebell; barbell; medicine ball; ankle band, pull-up bar

Dynamic Warm-up (see page 15)

Conditioning: Complete this circuit 1 time with as little rest as possible

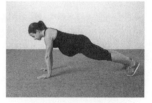

5 burpees or squat thrust–broad (mini) jumps > run 400 meters > 20-second rest and recover

10 burpees or squat thrust–broad (mini) jumps > run 300 meters > 20-second rest and recover

15 burpees or squat thrust–broad (mini) jumps > run 200 meters > 20-second rest and recover

BURPEE OR SQUAT THRUST–BROAD JUMPS

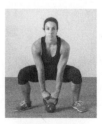

Strength Circuit (5 exercises): Complete this circuit 3 times

Exercise #1: Kettlebell Sumo Squat High Pull (Compound Movement)

Reps: 15

KETTLEBELL SUMO SQUAT HIGH PULL

Exercise #2: Barbell Push Jerk >
Inchworm Walkout (no push-up)
(Push and Core focus)

Reps: 15 Barbell Push Jerk immediately
into 10 Inchworm Walkouts—no rest
between exercises

Exercise #3: Medicine Ball Squat
Thrust, Throw, and Slam
(Compound Movement)

Reps: 10

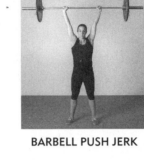

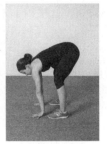

BARBELL PUSH JERK   **INCHWORM
WALKOUT
(NO PUSH-UP)**

Exercise #4: Snatch Grip BB Deadlift
(Bend focus)

Reps: 15

Exercise #5: Ankle Band Air Squats
(Squat focus)

Reps: 15

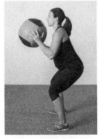

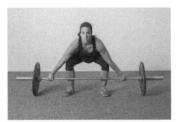

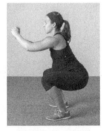

**MEDICINE BALL
SQUAT THRUST,
THROW, AND SLAM**

**SNATCH GRIP
BARBELL DEADLIFT**

**ANKLE BAND
AIR SQUATS**

Core: Tabata of Bent Legged V-ups and Forearm/Front Plank
Alternate between Bent Legged V-ups (BLV) and Planks: 20 seconds of BLV, rest 10
seconds; 20 seconds of forearm plank hold, rest 10 seconds. Repeat for 4 minutes.

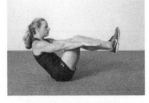

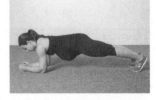

BENT LEGGED V-UPS   **FOREARM/FRONT PLANK**

Cool Down and Stretch:
Static stretch, mobility work, foam roller: Follow the Stretch Routine introduced on page 18.

Just Tying Your Sneakers . . . the New Workout!

Your Body Now

Strength	Lay off the *heavy* weight on squats and lifts.
Agility	Be careful! Many women feel clumsy, and it can be hard to see where you are stepping!
Stamina	You may be short of breath. Do what you can.
Well-being	Excitement and forgetfulness are common. Heartburn, constipation, and backaches continue.
Nutrition	Continue to take in 300 additional calories each day.
Modifications	Protect your pelvic ligaments from overstretching from bouncing (jogging) or impact (jumping).
Your baby now	The baby is the size of a honeydew melon, more than 18 inches from head to heel, weighing more than 5 pounds and packing on more than an ounce a day!

GETTING IT DONE

I fondly remember how much harder it was to put on socks and shoes during the last couple of months of pregnancy. Just finding my feet was hard! Working out every day was more of a mental challenge at this point but whenever I thought, "Why am I doing this?" I would just charge through and finish the workout no matter how ugly and uncomfortable it was. I knew the effort would pay off in the baby's health and my own well-being. And I didn't want to give up on myself and take it easy unless I had to. Besides, I still had a race to train for.

In the eighth month of my first pregnancy, with Steve's support and an approving nod from Dr. Heller, I signed up for a season-opening sprint-distance triathlon that was scheduled on Mother's Day, two weeks before my due date. In no way would this be an actual "race" for me. But I had a very good training base: I had been swimming in the pool all winter long, spinning, and riding my old mountain bike and road bike (with the biggest gel cushion seat I could find). I'd been doing strength training three or four days a week. So I figured, "Why not?" Steve was always with me on my outdoor bike rides and open water swims. Finding a wetsuit that

CHECKUP WITH DR. HELLER

Braxton-Hicks, or "painless uterine contractions" to distinguish them from the painful contractions associated with labor, can show up sporadically starting as early as twenty-four weeks. Many women mention them during their checkups. Should you be worried about them? What's normal?

A few Braxton-Hicks contractions per day are perfectly normal "practice" contractions. If you experience as many as four to six an hour, your practitioner may want to check by examination or ultrasound for any premature shortening of the cervix.

Braxton-Hicks contractions can respond to exercise, becoming more frequent with increased activity. An intestinal upset will also cause uterine irritability and set off more contractions, as will dehydration.

We have mentioned low blood pressure several times, but high blood pressure can be of concern in pregnancy as well. If you have high blood pressure before conceiving, then you probably manage it with diet and exercise (if you take medications, your physician will have prescribed a treatment that is safe during pregnancy). If you develop high blood pressure during pregnancy (gestational hypertension), it will probably resolve itself after delivery. In general, exercise helps control blood pressure. Rarely, though, severe hypertension starting in the second trimester can lead to preeclampsia, a condition that can be very dangerous to mother and baby. To guard against that, your health provider will check your blood pressure at every visit. If it is high enough to cause alarm (140/90), she will order tests to check for proteins in your urine. If preeclampsia is diagnosed, you may well get a prescription for bed rest. Staying still, lying on your left side, won't cure the condition, but it can help you continue the pregnancy until the baby is old enough to thrive after delivery.

continues

fits the pregnant body is challenging, to say the least. I suggest you borrow from several friends of different sizes until you find one that keeps you warm and dry.

Training went more smoothly in my second pregnancy, with Maddox. I had my sights set on the Buzzards Bay Sprint Triathlon early in my eighth month. I was still biking on my race bike and running . . . well I was still running enough to maintain a decent pace, believe it or not. Race day was picture perfect with great weather, ocean water temp, and atmosphere. As I walked around the race site, women noticed me and said, "Wow—You go, girl!" I did not have any expectations for my performance. Even though I was racing, the race was only against myself and the goal was to make it to the finish line.

continued

All in all, the third trimester can be a stressful time for mother and baby. Although most women and their babies sail through all nine months without any difficulties, there are a number of conditions that can arise that could impact an athlete's ability to continue to work out at what she perceives to be a normal level. In addition to hypertension, these include a serious fall causing fetal distress, or vaginal bleeding. Any of those medical complications could result in your physician suggesting that you curtail your activity. The most serious, such as bleeding or placenta previa, could even result in a prescription of bed rest for the remainder of the pregnancy. Even modified bed rest can be especially challenging for a woman who is normally very active, so be sure you and your family understand what is and is not allowed during this period.

Most women—and especially most athletes—have healthy, normal pregnancies. But it is important to remember that if your circumstances change, you should listen to your health care provider and follow his or her recommendations. If any of these following signs appear, immediately discontinue exercising and receive medical attention:

- Vaginal bleeding
- Prolonged dizziness or faintness
- Chest pain
- Persistent headache or out-of-the-ordinary muscle weakness
- Calf swelling or pain
- Uterine contractions
- Big decrease in fetal movement when you are inactive
- Fluid leaking from the vagina

Still, those little kudos gave me a big confidence boost that helped with my competitive drive and motivation.

The swim was very smooth, with the water nice and warm. There was plenty of room and no one kicked or bumped me. In transition I ripped off the wetsuit and hustled onto my bike and out of the transition area. I felt great on the bike! Doing so well in the swim and on the bike gave me the motivation to run the entire 5K even if I was uncomfortable. It was a really tough mental challenge to keep myself from walking until a woman turned as I was running by her and said, "Wow. I will not let a pregnant woman beat me." Huh, I thought. How rude. So I said, "Well you better get running faster, then." Okay, it's on. I would not stop and did my best to stick with her. I ended up just beating her out and finishing the race in 1:29:53, second place out of eleven Athena athletes! I have to say, out of all the races I have won or placed as an athlete, this was by far the toughest win and gave me the most amazing feeling of accomplishment because of the crazy physical, mental, and emotional challenges that I overcame.

WHAT'S GOING ON

Did you enjoy the past few months, when you were able to once again pass by a bathroom door without going in? After putting up with all the trips to the restroom the pressure on your bladder caused in the early months, you probably rejoiced when the uterus moved up into the abdomen—and off

> ### OLD WIVES' TALE: BATHING LATE IN PREGNANCY WILL CAUSE AN INFECTION OF THE AMNIOTIC FLUID.
>
> Don't be concerned that bathwater will travel up the vagina and cause an infection. Water doesn't travel up the vagina unless forced up by douching or jumping in a pool with your legs apart (go ahead, I dare you!). Even if some water does travel up the vagina, the cervical mucus plug protects the contents of the uterus. A nice warm bath can be very relaxing at this time—enjoy it!

your bladder—giving you some welcome relief. Now, in the third trimester, the weight of the uterus is on the bladder again and this time it's not kidding! During the last two months of pregnancy, almost all women notice increased urinary frequency and reduced bladder capacity, and sometimes even some leaking. Sneezing, coughing, laughing, maybe even just moving quickly can result in a little gush of pee. Of course, activities such as running, aerobics, lifting—in fact, most of the activities we talk about in this book—can cause you to leak. (Swimming is one exception to this rule—it's a bounce-free workout.) A belly band can reduce the pressure of the "bouncing ball" when you run; you can also wear a pad to catch any drips or do like I did and scope out the best bushes to slip behind or plan your route with a Dunkin' Donuts along the way. Avoid coffee, chocolates, spicy foods, and other foods that can irritate the bladder. Some women find that establishing a regular restroom schedule helps manage the situation. Kegels can improve the muscle tone of your pelvic floor, which also can make for a smoother labor and delivery (see page 89 for a refresher on Kegels). One more thing that can help: avoid getting constipated.

CONSTIPATION— SPACE IS TIGHT

Like heartburn, constipation only gets worse in late pregnancy. You may remember that in the early months, relaxin slowed the passage of food through your digestive system. This delay in gastric emptying and food processing gave your body extra time to extract the maximum nutrients for yourself and the baby. The hormonal action continues through your entire pregnancy, but in the third trimester its effect is compounded physically by the increasing size and weight of the uterus. The baby is pushing in all directions now. Pressure up on the stomach and upper abdomen makes reflux and heartburn even worse. And pressing down, it can effectively reduce the diameter of the bowel, leading to—you guessed it—constipation.

TIP: PACK YOUR HOSPITAL BAG!

During my first pregnancy, many people told me that because I worked out hard I would probably go into labor early. This led me to pack my hospital bag during Month 8. Of course, by Month 9, most of it had been unpacked so I could use it! For my second, the hospital bag never got packed, due to my procrastination and overconfidence that I was in control.

Here are the things to be sure to pack:

- camera
- stopwatch/chrono watch (it's fun to time the contractions)
- flip-flops or nonslip socks/booties (you won't want to sit still)
- comfortable clothes for a few days, just in case
- toiletries
- chocolate
- some magazines
- baby stuff . . .

Here's what *not* to pack:

- tubing or other exercise equipment

This is the big event you have been training for. As far as I was concerned, once labor was over I planned to enjoy a little recovery time!

GET READY FOR LIFE WITH BABY

The first month or so after you bring the baby home, your schedule will definitely not be your own! Face it, you'll be tired and sleep deprived. You'll be busy, taking care of the baby and maybe dealing with the logistics of breast-feeding, an even bigger challenge if you don't want to do it in public. You may not have easy access to daycare, and even if your gym offers daycare, it might not accept infants younger than six weeks. But if you're ready and want to get in a workout, a little planning now will make things easier after you deliver:

- Get a running stroller—The newest ones have three big air-filled tires to cover mixed terrain. Look for good cornering ability and a deep, comfortable seat for Junior. Be sure the stroller has a safety strap so you don't lose hold of it! When the weather is fine, you and baby can get a nice run in. Bring some tubing and leg bands and create your own outdoor boot camp workout.
- Make sure you've got the right gym. Check with your gym on their daycare policies, and confirm that it offers extended hours. If they do, you can squeeze in a workout at 5:00 a.m. while your partner stays home snoozing with the baby (if they're lucky!).
- Shop now for your postdelivery workout needs. Even if you have a gym membership, set up a mini home gym with some weights and tubing for days when it just doesn't work to go out. Find an old spinning bicycle or dust off your treadmill. Check the equipment list (page 20) and fill in any gaps.
- Start looking for a pediatrician who will suit your lifestyle and whose office hours fit your schedule.
- Prep and freeze some casseroles and meals. You'll be so happy to find them in the freezer after the baby is born!

The solution? You probably guessed that, too: grazing on complex carbohydrates and staying well hydrated.

All in all, things are getting pretty crowded in your abdomen, and the baby is feeling the squeeze, too. One of the great joys of pregnancy is feeling the baby move. The baby is still moving up to thirty times an hour, but by the eighth month there's less room in the baby's gym. You might notice less "full-body fitness" activity, but you will still feel plenty of smaller pokes and kicks, especially at night. Some women notice that their babies move less after their workouts, and this concerns them. Now is the time to do a little grazing with a high-quality snack; the increase in your blood sugar will give your baby a rush of energy. If you are ever worried that your baby has stopped moving, Dr. Heller advises having something to eat and then lying down on your left side, putting your hand on your belly to feel the movements. If you have been keeping track of your baby's normal activity patterns, that will help you judge when a change is significant. Of course, if the baby is truly not moving for an unusually long period of time, call your health care provider, who can check your baby's heart rate and movements.

Toward the end of pregnancy, the mother slows or even stops adding fat, and a higher percentage of the nutrients goes to support the baby's growth. This is a big growth phase for the baby, who is adding up to a pound a week toward the end. Continue to take in only about 300 calories above the amount that maintained your prepregnancy weight to ensure that the baby gets what it needs and nothing more. Make them high-quality foods and *try* not to give in too much to your temptations for jelly doughnuts (guilty!), cheese steak subs (guilty!), or Jim Dandy Sundaes (guilty again!). If you succumb to

"I was so buoyant—but really not in a helpful way. It's like having a basketball on your stomach. I'm not usually a really buoyant person, but I could float with my hands and feet out of the water. After watching me do the breast stroke, my husband said, 'The way you hit the water, your belly *actually pushes you backward.*' It was like a shelf. But I was able to do flip turns the entire time!"

—KATE, SWIMMER, MOTHER OF ONE

the urge to take in too many extra calories at this time, it can and will lead to a bigger, fatter baby. One thing for sure—you will have less impulse control, so put the sweets out of sight. When you really want them, make the trip to get them . . . or have your partner do it for you!

Around the eighth month is when you truly grasp the fact your life is going to change forever. That belly is huge and getting bigger every day; suddenly you realize: there is no turning back. If you have not finished putting the crib together or any other baby room preparations, now is the time to get it done. As far as being there for your partner and supporting your lovely pregnant bride, these are the weeks when you want to be extra supportive without being pushy. This could be challenging. Depending on how the wind was blowing, my encouraging comments were seen as supportive or too demanding. It also didn't help that I sometimes made stupid "reflex" comments. It was fantastic and inspiring to see her work out so hard, still pushing more weight and getting more done than nonpregnant athletes. But my enthusiasm for her ability would get in the way when, for example, she asked me to pick up a spoon that had fallen onto the kitchen floor. My ill-fated response? "Honey, you just did all that lifting and now you can't pick up a little spoon—come on!" Talk about a brain fart.

Steve

Your hormones still have a few more tricks in store for you. Estrogen levels increase throughout pregnancy before dropping sharply at birth. You may start to have hot flashes as your hormone levels fluctuate. Deal with these the same way you deal with hot weather: dress in layers and stay hydrated. Most hot flashes only last 10 to 15 seconds, but if you are "always hot," sit near a fan.

CATCHING YOUR BREATH

No matter what type of athlete you are or what your cardio routine is, you'll probably notice that it's harder to catch your breath as the expanding uterus crowds your diaphragm and lungs. Despite your difficulty breathing, you are actually taking in more oxygen and using it more efficiently that you

> "I rowed on the water every day while I was pregnant. Running and cycling didn't work at all after the fifth month, but I could row right up to the end."
>
> —MARY, ROWER, MOTHER OF TWO

did before you got pregnant. It just seems harder. This sensation that you need to breathe more deeply will subside when the baby drops (two or three weeks before delivery for first babies).

For now, you can't work at your old pace, but give yourself a personal challenge—set a goal that will motivate you to stay strong. Training for a race—even one I didn't plan to win—gave me something to shoot for and kept my mind *off* the discomfort of training and *on* the huge goal I had just set. I told

PREGNANT OLYMPIANS

We may think that pregnant Olympians are a recent phenomenon, but over the years, more than a dozen women are known to have competed while pregnant. The earliest on record was Swedish skater Magda Julin who took home the gold when she was three months pregnant at the 1920 Games. In 1952, American diver Juno Stover-Irwin medaled at three and a half months.

Confident that the baby is safely tucked in the protective muscles and fluid of the uterus, athletes have even competed in handball (Anna-Marie Johansson, 2012), volleyball (Kerri Walsh Jennings, gold, 2012), and equestrian (Anky van Grunsven, gold, 2004). Two different German athletes competed in the skeleton event (Diana Sartor, 2010, and Kerstin Szymkowiak, silver, 2010)—each was in her third month, so I guess they weren't having problems with nausea!

The 2012 Olympics saw at least two pregnant athletes, one at each end of the pregnancy calendar: Kerri Walsh Jennings noticed her pregnancy days before the Games (see page 45), and Malaysian sport shooter Nur Survani Mohd Taibi was thirty-four weeks along.

myself that if I wasn't up to racing on race day, then I wouldn't do it; I would just cheer Steve on from the sidelines. I would encourage any and all pregnant athletes to shoot for a race goal if you are feeling good and have a healthy pregnancy. Don't even think about your past race times. . . . This race is *not* an opportunity to compare old stats. And don't bother with traveling to a destination race—you won't do well and most doctors advise against flying after thirty-six weeks anyway. Just be happy that you are out there and able to do something like this in your last weeks of pregnancy! Set a goal, work toward it, do your best, and have fun.

Gradually move to low-impact activities. But keep working out—women who exercise through the third trimester have the greatest benefits: less fat gain for mother and baby, smoother labor and delivery, faster recovery.

THE IMPORTANCE OF YOUR CORE

Do you feel as if you have a bowling ball taped to your belly? It takes strong abdominal muscles to support it, cantilevered out there. I am sure you have been keeping up your core strength so your lower back and abs can do their jobs, helping you maintain your posture and avoid backaches (nearly impossible in Months 8 and 9 but worth trying). Those same strong abs will assist the uterus in delivery and help make you one hell of a pusher to get that baby out. The stronger your abs (especially the transverse abs) and pelvic floor muscles, the longer and harder you will be able to push. I came to discover that this is *very important*, and it helped make my deliveries very quick.

The consequences of not working your core can lead to more low back and upper back discomfort and a more taxing delivery. In addition, it's possible for the outward pressure of the uterus to split the linea alba (the vertical sheath dividing the abdominal muscles) in late pregnancy, causing backaches now and after delivery. This is much more likely to happen if the abdominals are weak, so keep up your core work.

Above all, listen closely to your body and monitor your exertion level during this month's workouts and any races you enter. You are an experienced athlete, so recognize and respect your limits. Here is one of my workout plans from Month 8.

Sunday	Monday	Tuesday	Wednesday	Thursday	Friday	Saturday
Off	Morning run, strength; evening bike if feeling up to it	Morning run; evening swim	Morning bike, strength	Morning track run; evening swim	Morning short run if up to it, strength	Morning strength and/or morning swim, bike, and/or run (a brick workout) based on how I am feeling

MONTH 8 SAMPLE STRENGTH WORKOUT

Suggested modifications for Month 8: In the eighth month, stay on both feet for exercises that you previously did on single legs. Be sure to stay close to a support for extra balance—for example, if you do Donkey Calf Raises, stand close to something you can hold on to if you need it. At this point sprinting is a thing of the past, so replacing that with jogging shouldn't be an issue. The most important thing is just being able to keep moving and getting through your workouts the best you can.

If you do not have a training partner, consider moving to indoor cycling to accommodate your lack of balance. Balance is not an issue with a recumbent bike or ERG/rower, and it will be more comfortable on the tush!

If you run, wear clothing that is supportive (spandexlike materials) as well as a running support belt and a strong/supportive sports bra. All of these products help with compression, keeping things in place and helping you feel more comfortable while moving. Use the elliptical trainer or a treadmill if the roads are becoming too much for the joints or you are not feeling confident navigating outdoor obstacles such as curbs, pot holes, or ice.

If aerobics is your preferred activity, skip the jumps now.

The Workout

Equipment needed: Pull-up bar; dumbbells; barbell; rower

Dynamic Warm-up (see page 15)

Conditioning: 5-minute AMRAP (as many reps as possible)
Complete as many repetitions of 5 Pull-ups, then 10 Push-ups, then 15 Squats as possible in 5 minutes

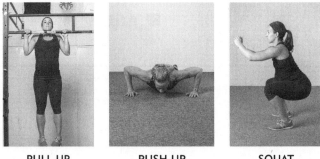

PULL-UP   PUSH-UP   SQUAT

Strength Circuit (4 exercises): Complete this circuit 2 times

Exercise #1: Dumbbell Single-arm Bicep Curl to Overhead Press (Compound Movement)

Reps: 10 per side

Exercise #2: Dumbbell Front Squat > Forward Quarter Lunge (Squat and Lunge focus)

Reps: Complete 1 Dumbbell Front Squat, then 1 Quarter Lunge—repeat sequence 10 times

Exercise #3: Dumbbell Farmer's Carry (Conditioning focus)

Reps: 50 yards

Exercise #4: Donkey Calf Raises (Push focus)

Reps: 20

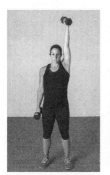 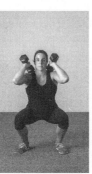 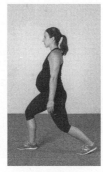 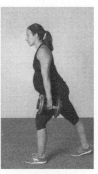 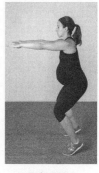

| DUMBBELL SINGLE-ARM BICEP CURL TO OVERHEAD PRESS | DUMBBELL FRONT SQUAT | FORWARD QUARTER LUNGE | DUMBBELL FARMER'S CARRY | DONKEY CALF RAISES |

Conditioning: 250 meter row > 10 Dumbbell Thrusters > 20 Bent-leg V-ups

Reps: 3 times through with 30-second recovery between sets

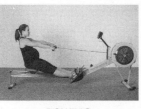 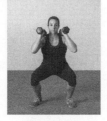 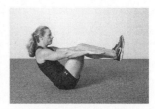

| ROWING | DUMBBELL THRUSTERS | BENT-LEG V-UPS |

Cool Down and Stretch:

Static stretch, mobility work, foam roller: Follow the Stretch Routine introduced on page 18.

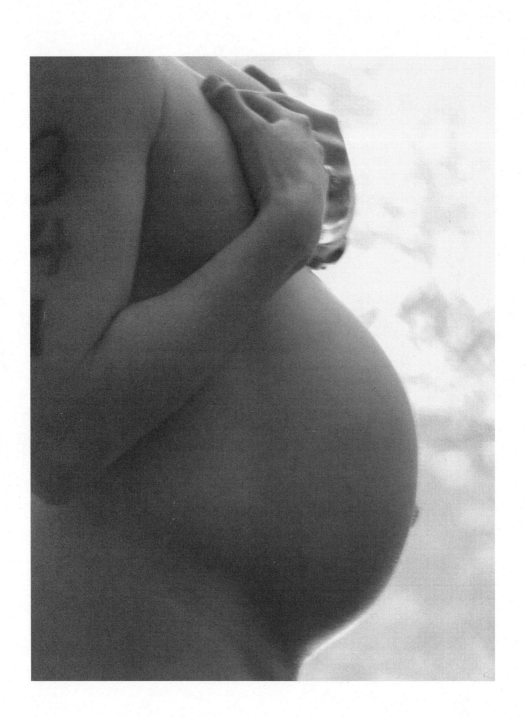

The Longest Mile, or Maybe Five

Your Body Now

Strength	Work on your upper body and arms. Keep squatting—don't go low—squats will help with labor.
Agility	Be careful—your hands are swollen, your joints are wobbly, and you can't see your feet!
Stamina	You're probably short of breath; everything seems hard.
Well-being	With the finish line in sight, you may have extra energy this month. Your emotions will probably be a combination of impatience, irritability, and excitement.
Nutrition	Maintain 300 calories over your prepregnancy intake; don't let your workouts create a calorie deficit.
Modifications	Recognize that your balance is off—stay on both feet and off the Bosu ball. Curtail anaerobic work such as sprints.
Your baby now	Your little punkin' is as big as a pumpkin, 20 inches, 7.6 pounds! Fully developed, even the lungs are ready to go.

The final few weeks are definitely the toughest in every way—physically, mentally, and emotionally. By day you may be moody, irritable, and tired. By night, you have to deal with heartburn, the just plain awkwardness of the belly, and a slew of new sleep challenges. Face it, just getting out of bed is no fun, let alone getting through workouts. If this is your second or third baby, you may feel this even more strongly, because your muscles and ligaments started out more stretched and relaxed and now they have to work even harder to support you. Even if you feel pretty good, you are counting off those mile markers—Week 35, Week 36, Week 37, . . .

This is when you hope those old wives' tales about exercise triggering labor might be true. I don't know about you, but I did everything I could think of to induce labor in the final weeks. I worked out consistently, adding stair repeats at the local hospital and hill repeats at the longest local hill, as well as indulging in more spicy food and sex. And I raced in the ninth month of both pregnancies. All these were supposed to speed things along, right? Guess again.

Your workouts this month are by far the hardest to get through mentally and emotionally, if you make it this far! I had my days of "Why?!" but I had more days of "Wow, I did it and I feel great."

TOO EXCITED—OR UNCOMFORTABLE—TO SLEEP?

Plenty of factors, including that huge belly, contribute to the sleeplessness that many women report in the last weeks of pregnancy. On the emotional side, you might be excited about the baby, or having some totally understandable anxiety about the changes in store for you and your family. Physically, you are still dealing with many of the challenges of early pregnancy, only more so! For example, the pressure of the uterus on your stomach combines with relaxin's loosening effect on the esophageal sphincter to make heartburn even worse than it was earlier. Sleeping with your head elevated may help,

> ## OLD WIVES' TALE: RUNNING WILL CAUSE THE MEMBRANE TO BREAK.
>
> Sorry, no. The repetitive foot strike of running and jumping of aerobics do not cause the membranes to break before the onset of labor. Even after the mouth of the cervix has begun to dilate, these activities do not trigger premature delivery, although they can make you very uncomfortable and stress your pelvic ligaments.
>
> But remember that, according to Dr. Joseph Clapp's research, regular exercisers do tend to deliver five to seven days earlier than nonexercisers, have shorter labors, and fewer medical interventions such as episiotomies, induction, or pain relief.

and remember Dr. Heller's advice to take an antacid or other heartburn reliever (see pages 64 and 87). And as the baby hogs more and more space and presses on your bladder, you'll be making more nighttime trips to the bathroom, too.

A couple of new problems complete the list of bedtime complaints. First, just getting comfortable is a challenge. The best position for sleeping is on your left side because it keeps the weight of the uterus off the vein returning blood to your heart and allows the best blood flow to the placenta and your kidneys. This improves your body's ability to eliminate wastes and fluids (and so helps reduce swelling in your feet and hands). If you sleep on your back, the weight of the baby on your organs and spine can reduce circu-

CHECKUP WITH DR. HELLER

While most women are more than ready for their babies to be born after nine months of pregnancy, unless you have actually scheduled a delivery by cesarean or induction it is almost impossible to predict when the baby will arrive. But there are some clues that will help you recognize the baby's impending arrival.

First, the baby will drop lower in your pelvis. You may not feel the actual movement, but you are likely to notice its effects: greater lung and abdominal capacity and increased pressure on the bladder. If this is your first pregnancy, this dropping can take place as early as several weeks before labor; in subsequent pregnancies, the baby doesn't usually drop until labor begins.

Your body will pass the mucus plug that has sealed your cervical canal during the pregnancy. This may show as a brown or bloody discharge or an actual plug of thick mucus. This may happen as much as a few days before labor.

The Braxton-Hicks contractions that you have been experiencing for several months now will intensify and become more frequent. As your contractions become longer and closer together, the sac of amniotic fluid may break. This is usually a sign that labor has begun.

If your amniotic sac breaks or your contractions are frequent and regular (as many as eight) for an hour, call your medical provider and go to the hospital or birthing center.

lation and make back pain and hemorrhoids more likely, and who needs that? Your back is already going to feel tired and worked, so do anything you can to help ease the pain. Turn on your left side, and put a pillow between your knees and other pillows around you to make yourself more comfortable. A body pillow between my legs was a huge help. Don't feel bad kicking your partner out of bed to make room for the pillows (in fact, your partner may be happy for an excuse to sleep somewhere else to get away from your snoring!). Wearing a bra at night will support your breasts; you may even want to sleep in a maternity belt.

Working out should reduce the chance of leg cramps, but they can still be a problem. Cramps may be caused by the extra 30-or-so pounds your legs are toting around all day, every day, or they may be a result of diminished blood return to the heart. Either way, keeping your training up should help you avoid them. Keep your knees slightly bent when you stand and avoid locking them out (which inhibits blood return). Remember to stay well hydrated even though you really don't want to because of the bathroom trips. Some people report that a few calf stretches or rolling your calves on a foam roller or hard ball (such as a lacrosse ball or baseball) before bed can reduce the severity and frequency of leg cramps.

To top off your sleeping challenges, you'll probably notice that the baby gets active around the time you are ready to call it a night. Your normal movements during the day tend to soothe the baby; when you stop "rocking" and go to bed, the baby wakes up. Besides that, you are quieter and more likely to notice the baby's activity than when you are moving around yourself. Mackenzie and Maddox were very active at night and often got the hiccups. That felt really weird the first time, but I loved it after I learned it was only hiccups and not a problem!

Finally, just as you drift off, you'll notice that you need to run to the bathroom—again—and the whole process starts over!

Even though these issues in themselves are nothing to worry about, being overly tired physically, mentally, and emotionally can definitely interfere with your workout plans. Even if you can't sleep, be sure to get plenty of rest. Put your feet up—this might be a challenge if you're keeping your head elevated, too! Some women find that taking a walk can help. If you are not able to continue your routine, walking is very relaxing and soothes the baby. Just be sure you have a safe, flat, well-lit environment.

As the partner of a pregnant athlete, you may or may not put your own athletic pursuits on hold to help support the mother of your child, but I felt the best way to support Brandi was to train and race alongside her. As you make those decisions of whether or not to train and race with your partner, consider a few tidbits of info I learned the hard way.

1. Her hormones, her excitement, and stress of racing will definitely impact her mood. You will undoubtedly need to be more patient and relaxed on race day or leading up to it and be as supportive as possible. That may include encouraging remarks on how great she has been doing and how well she will do. You can reduce her worries and stress by getting her race gear ready.

2. She may be self-conscious about performing while pregnant. This could come from how she thinks she look ("big," especially if it's later in their pregnancy), but also how she thinks others might be thinking about or might say when they see a pregnant woman racing. Be prepared to "defend" her from comments such as, "How can you put your child at risk?" "Are you that selfish that you can't give this up?" Understand that outside the athletic community, people don't all understand the science behind the benefits of activity and exercise for the baby as well as the mother. As you may be wasting your breath trying to convince others in that fleeting moment, focus on her. Tell her that what she is doing is the best thing she can be doing for your baby and you are so proud of her.

Steve

DAYTIME CHALLENGES

Once you climb out of bed, another thing that might slow you down is being short of breath—like heartburn, a combination of hormonal effects and the position of the baby. If you feel breathless, just do what you can. Remember to gauge your effort by perceived exertion—not by your heart rate (which may seem low for the amount of work you are doing) or especially by comparing yourself to what you used to do! That is all a thing of the past, so just be happy that you are still able to exercise. You'll get your wind back when the baby drops later this month if this is your first. When the baby drops, or descends lower in the pelvis, your lungs will have more room—you'll be able to catch your breath and you may have less heartburn. On the other hand, your bladder will be even more cramped and your pelvis will feel even more weighed down. (Second and subsequent babies usually don't drop until labor.)

Another benefit of the baby dropping is that your stomach gets a little more room. Until then, it doesn't seem fair—at last morning sickness is behind you and you're ravenous all the time, but you cannot eat even a moderate-size meal. Not only will it not fit into your squished tummy, but it will also most likely give you heartburn! The best thing you can do at this point is eat smaller meals, more often, to help you take in enough extra calories without staying up all night with an upset stomach or starving an hour after each meal.

> "I'll come out and say it: I hated being pregnant. I felt like something was taking over my body. I never got sick, in fact I was very healthy. But I didn't enjoy the experience. I just felt *big*. But labor and delivery—that's another story. That was great, almost like an adventure race."
>
> —CAROL, TRIATHLETE, MOTHER OF TWO

Breakfast: cereal or oatmeal with fruit and milk; half peanut butter sandwich

Snack: yogurt or cottage cheese and fruit; handful of nuts

Lunch: soup and sandwich, fruit

Snack: crackers and fruit, milk or hot chocolate

Supper: a light and delicious healthy meal, such as chicken and a salad

If you are following a vegan diet, try a soy smoothie with lots of fruit. Eat nuts and other high-fat choices to ensure proper weight gain; supplement iron, calcium, and other nutrients as your practitioner recommends, and use iodized salt. If you are eating a Paleo or gluten-free plan, be sure to take in enough complex carbs.

HIGH-OCTANE ENERGY

You may be pleasantly surprised by big bursts of energy in the ninth month. I've heard that many women have an urge to clean, tidy the house, and paint the nursery. Increased adrenalin and emotions both contribute to this "nesting" urge. You'll probably welcome the return of your energy with open arms, but don't overdo it with any heavy weights or risky moves. I got lucky, and during my early morning workouts I always felt ready for whatever was in the training plan. But because of my changing center of gravity, I had to be mindful of everything I was doing at every minute of the workout. And even though I was paying attention, I had a couple of eye-opening experiences. After I almost took a tumble while using an ankle band, I learned to think twice and find modifications that would make every exercise safer for my baby and me.

The fact that you might deliver a baby any day now is no reason to veg out—but keep in mind that it's okay to relax. Remember to listen to your body and be ready to modify or even abandon your planned workout for the day, depending on how you feel. But it helps to have a goal, and for each pregnancy I had a race goal in the last month to help keep my mind off the misery and discomfort of pregnancy as well as to have another reason to stick with my daily exercise routine. With Mackenzie it was the Hopkinton Season Opener Sprint Triathlon, on Mother's Day, two weeks before my due date—the perfect day to deliver my first baby! Nevertheless, even though I had my heart set on doing this triathlon, I knew that if I did not feel up to it, I wouldn't do it.

With Maddox I was running up until the end so I decided to run the local Turkey Trot 5-Miler four days before my due date.

> "I was planning to do an open water swim on New Year's Eve. I had been joking that my birth plan was to step in the ocean just outside Boston and then go straight to the hospital. That didn't happen—he was born on December 28. He was probably thinking, 'I hear what you're saying out there and you're *crazy*, so I'm coming out early!'"
>
> —KATE, SWIMMER, MOTHER OF ONE

Steve pushed Mackenzie in the stroller and I threw on my Home Depot utility belt with suspender straps to keep everything tight. When the gun went off and I started out, I felt great, keeping in mind that "great" is relative! I felt pregnant and ready to burst, but I could shuffle along with a nice trot. I developed a cycle: get into a good rhythm, start to cramp, slow down, walk for a couple of minutes, then start to jog again. This run was way more of a mental challenge than the triathlon. It was a long 5 miles of shuffling and waddling but in the end I got it done. My belly was huge—so huge that it crossed the finish line long before the rest of me! I was able to relax the rest of the day.

PREPARING FOR THE BIG DAY

Although about a third of women in the United States today have their babies by cesarean, most athletes opt for vaginal delivery if they can. After all, a cesarean, although easier in some respects than vaginal labor

RACE DAY, MAY 11, 2008

What an amazing morning! I was feeling really pregnant and ready to get this triathlon done. Of course, I felt like a beached whale in my wetsuit, but I didn't care. I had a smooth swim and when I reached the beach I was in race mode. Usually I block out people cheering and yelling as it is all background noise to me, but that day I heard a women scream at the top of her lungs, "You go, girl! Damn, you are pregnant! Wow, go get it done!" I never looked at her but I heard her loud and clear. She made my race day. She gave me a boost of energy, confidence, and adrenaline to get me going and keep me focused.

Wetsuit off, I plopped down on the ground to get my bike shoes on. No way could I do that standing up! I was working so hard just to put on my shoes, it was hysterical. I threw on my cycling helmet and started running out of transition, making a flying hop onto my bike seat. This bike course is hilly—my toughest challenge through both pregnancies—but I just kept pedaling and going as hard as I could. After the ride, I got off the bike and jogged back into transition to get my sneakers on and send my relay runner out on the course. I opted for a 1.5-mile run instead of the full 5K because I had pelvic pain while running during my first pregnancy. Jeremee (my running teammate) and I ended up winning the team relay category with a time of 1:18:26.

Steve had quite a different experience that day. Here's how he tells the story.

The Season Opener Sprint Triathlon in southern Massachusetts is a great race with a fun course and a fantastic way to start our race season off together each year. But this was the first time Brandi would be competing in a race being this pregnant, so I was a bit on edge. As this is an early season race, the water temperature would be quite cold—low 60s to upper 50s—and the shock of the water temperature alone would prove to be too much for many swimmers. But after a warm-up swim I was confident that she would be fine.

I did, however, have my greatest scare of both pregnancies during this race. I was about 8 miles into the bike portion of my race, a state cruiser blew by me with its lights and sirens going, followed by a fire truck and then an ambulance. Thoughts of terror raced through my mind—"She went into labor" or worse. By the time I rode back to the transition area I was in a panic and I ran up to the race director to find out what went wrong. I was so relieved to learn that all the commotion was not for Brandi, but for an older man who had a heart attack during the swim, due to the cold temp. I gave the director a big hug with a huge smile on my face and carried on for the run potion of the race. It was not until later that day that I felt bad about feeling so good that this poor man had a heart attack and needed medical assistance and not my wife!

and delivery, is abdominal surgery and dictates a four- to six-week recovery period. After vaginal delivery, you could be up and around in a few days. (I don't say you'll be frisky, but you will be moving!)

Even if you plan to have your baby the old fashioned way, you'll want to educate yourself about both delivery methods during the ninth month. There are medical reasons (such as high blood pressure or problems with the placenta) that might indicate that a C-section is the best delivery route for your baby after all. If your baby presents as a breech delivery or other complications arise during labor and delivery, you may have to have a cesarean without having a choice. No matter which delivery route your baby or body ends up choosing, a strong abdomen and pelvic floor will help, so keep up your core and Kegel exercises. Having a cesarean once meant all your subsequent babies would have to be born that way, but this is no longer true. Many women choose VAC (vaginal after cesarean) delivery for their next child. So pack your bags and make your preparations with some flexibility in mind, and get used to the idea that the baby's vote counts more than yours does.

THE DAY YOU'VE BEEN WAITING FOR

Finally, the day you have spent the past nine months preparing for will arrive and you will go into labor. You may have been having contractions for a while, but now they are longer, stronger, and closer together, and

> "The birth of my daughter, Isla, hasn't lessened my enjoyment of running, or my desire to win. I'm just as committed, if not more so, because there's someone else to run for."
>
> —PAULA RADCLIFFE, CURRENT WORLD-RECORD HOLDER IN THE MARATHON

nothing you do—eating, moving around, staying still—changes them. You have a brownish discharge or pass your mucus plug, your water breaks.

If you go past your due date, your medical team may decide to induce labor. For Mackenzie we scheduled a time with Dr. Heller to induce me. We went in about midmorning and walked laps all day while the pitocin kicked in. All in all, we walked 40 laps around the hospital wing. The nurses were timing my splits, no kidding. Finally at about 3:30 p.m. Dr. Heller checked the dilation and said I was ready to have my water broken. At that moment I went into labor and started having contractions. My nurse, Dido, encouraged me to try anything and everything to get through the contractions and help move things along. We progressed from the wall, to the physioball, to the bathtub, then onto the toilet, then near the bed and finally onto the bed to start pushing. I was lucky not to have extreme back pain (back labor), but some women find that getting on all fours or having their partner massage their back between contractions helps with this. Finally, while my legs were in the air, my nurse screamed at me to teach me how to push, and I mean really *push*. "When you think you can't push anymore, give one more push," she told me. At 7:00 p.m. on the nose, Mackenzie popped out. Those three hours were the most painful of my life, but I kept pushing. Pain would come and go, but it was bearable and I didn't have to opt for the drugs.

With Maddox, my water broke at home about 9:45 p.m. When we told the doctor the contractions were about four or five minutes apart, she said, "You better come in now." We arrived at the hospital and things moved pretty quickly. Unlike Dido, my first nurse who had thirty years' experience and didn't mind yelling at me, this nurse was shy and soft-spoken. I needed her to speak louder so I could hear her over my pain screams and breathing. Steve recognized my frustration and stepped in, asked her to move aside, and started coaching me, which meant encouraging me to keep pushing even when I thought I couldn't anymore. This kept me on track. After about an hour and a half, Maddox graced us with his presence.

Once you go into labor, it's as if the starting gun has sounded for a long, challenging event. You've been here before—well, maybe not here *exactly*, but you know how to push yourself, and you know how to work through pain. If you've been in childbirth classes, you've been practicing breathing. Find a breathing rhythm now, just like in an event, and use your breath to push yourself through the pain. All my ab work and intense training certainly helped give me the strength to push beyond my limits and get those babies out of my body fast.

RUNNING ON FUMES

If you want to give your pelvic ligaments a break this month, target your upper body (chest, upper back, core, biceps, and triceps). But don't totally neglect your pelvic floor. And while you may not get as low as you used to, you need to keep squatting. Just do what you can. Even if you don't squat during labor and delivery (as many women around the world do), it will strengthen your core and lower body. You'll thank me later when you push that baby out fast. While you wait for your big day, this chapter's workout recognizes that your ligaments are loose, your belly is huge, your balance is chancy, and you are running on mental willpower! Literally.

Sunday	Monday	Tuesday	Wednesday	Thursday	Friday	Saturday
Off	Morning run, strength	Morning run; evening swim	Morning bike, strength	Morning run, swim if feeling good.	Morning run if up to it, strength	Morning strength

MONTH 9 SAMPLE STRENGTH WORKOUT

Suggested modifications for Month 9: In the ninth month, don't do Bosu (or other instability-inducing) push-ups. If you do any push-ups, you may even want to modify them and do them from your knees (yes, this is hard for me to admit, but if I had high reps, I would do them modified). Stay on both feet (no single-leg balances or step-ups), and don't do lateral tosses or any other lateral stress moves. You have probably already cut way back on the running—if not, good for you if you can keep it up! I still ran, just cut down on the volume (and the intensity took care of itself). You'll get your sprints and anaerobic work done just by walking up the stairs or doing hill repeats trying to induce labor.

If none of your usual workouts appeals to you, consider recumbent rowing. You will stay cooler because your motion on the seat will "fan" you. Rowing is impact-free and takes the weight off your feet and legs. The rower may not be a common piece of equipment in many facilities because it takes up a lot of floor space. It's a challenging exercise, but for those who can't or shouldn't run and don't have access to a aerodyne bike, the ERG/rower is your next best choice to give the entire body a fantastic workout.

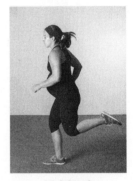

JOGGING

The Workout

Equipment needed: Dumbbells; barbell; physioball

Dynamic Warm-up: (see page 15)

Conditioning: Waddle fast/light jog 50 yards, 10 Air Squats, easy walk back 6 times

Strength Circuit (6 exercises): Complete this circuit 3 times

Exercise #1: Barbell Back Squat (Squat focus)
Reps: 15

Exercise #2: Wide-grip Push-up (Careful of the belly!) (Push focus)
Reps: 10

Exercise #3: Physioball Single-arm Incline Chest Press (Push focus)
Reps: 10 per arm

Exercise #4: Physioball or Bench Dumbbell Skull Crusher (Push focus)
Reps: 15

Exercise #5: Bird Dogs (Core focus)
Reps: 10 per side

Exercise #6: Physioball Double-Leg Hamstring Bridges into Physioball Hamstring Curls (Pull focus)
Reps: 20/20

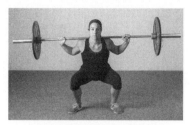

BARBELL BACK SQUAT

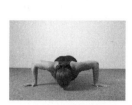

WIDE-GRIP PUSH-UP

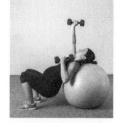

PHYSIOBALL SINGLE-ARM
INCLINE CHEST PRESS

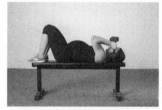

PHYSIOBALL OR BENCH
DUMBBELL SKULL CRUSHER

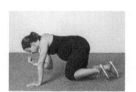

BIRD DOGS

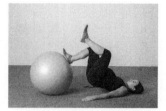

PHYSIOBALL HAMSTRING
CURLS

Conditioning: Waddle/jog fast 50 yards, 5 Air Squats, easy walk back 6 times

Cool Down and Stretch:
   Static stretch, mobility work, foam roller: Follow the Stretch Routine introduced on page 18.

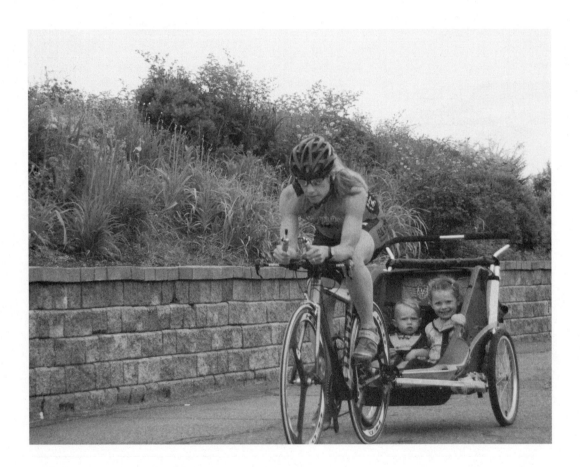

Back on Track, Back to Fit

Your Body Now

Strength	Your uterus is enlarged and still heavy. Lay off any heavy lifting, sit-ups, or anything that strains the pelvic floor.
Agility	You will still have some joint laxity and your center of gravity is still forward because of the enlarged uterus.
Stamina	Some fatigue is normal. If you had a C-section, expect to feel tired for at least six weeks.
Well-being	Most women feel good, although a period of baby blues is normal, as are some hormonal-based mood swings. Studies show that exercising can speed both physical and emotional recovery.
Nutrition	Return to prepregnancy caloric levels if you are not breast-feeding (eat more if you are breast-feeding), and concentrate on good nutrition. Stay hydrated. Complex carbs will help any constipation.
Modifications	Be careful to avoid abdominal strain. Be attentive to joint instability, which can cause injuries. Avoid jumping and high-impact exercises.

Congratulations! You've reached the finish line! There is no better feeling in the world than hearing your baby cry for the first time after that last hard push. I hope that you experienced a smooth and uncomplicated delivery. Every delivery is different and anything can happen, so as much as I "trained" for giving birth to my two amazing children, I didn't go to the hospital expecting it to be easy, painless, or quick. I had prepared myself for anything by having no expectations or setting my heart on any particular methods. Even though I wanted to go "natural," I had nothing against taking drugs or painkillers if I needed them, and man did I come close! But I wanted to see how much pain I could tolerate before giving in and screaming, "Give me all the drugs you've got—*now*!" That was my mental and physical challenge during that event: how hard could I push and how much could I take for how long, before giving in or reaching the finish line of getting these babies out of my body? Of course, hindsight is 20/20 and now that they are running around like wild animals it would have been much easier to keep them safely trapped in my body for their entire lives.

After Mackenzie (baby #1), I felt as if I been hit by a truck! Every muscle in my body was sore from pushing so hard, thanks to Dido, my amazing delivery room nurse who knew I could give a little bit more even when I thought I was done and felt like I was going to die. Still, both my deliveries were relatively short and easy—and at least some of the credit must go to all that abdominal, squat, and deadlift work during the pregnancy. Mackenzie, from water break to delivery took four hours—pretty unheard of for an induced delivery. Maddox was even quicker. From water break at home, to drive to the hospital, to labor and delivery was about two hours. After Maddox was in my hands and all was said and done, the doctor turned to me and said, "If every delivery was like yours, my job would be a piece of cake." That comment, combined of course with delivering a very healthy little boy, really made my night! I hope yours goes as well!

OLD WIVES' TALE: REGULAR EXERCISE DURING BREAST-FEEDING DECREASES THE QUANTITY AND SPOILS THE TASTE OF BREAST MILK.

This is indeed true—for *dairy* cows! Luckily, human mothers don't experience the same effects. Studies now show that frequent, sustained, moderate-to-high-intensity running does not impair the quantity or quality of breast milk.

The concern over the taste of the milk is because—at least for those dairy cows—exercise increased the amount of lactic acid in the milk, giving it a sour taste that the calves rejected. But the studies showed that exercise did not change the human babies' nursing behavior—so the taste was probably not affected.

BACK TO IT

How you deliver, the medications you receive, and the length of your labor will all greatly affect how you feel and how long it takes to recover after you pop the baby out. After the excitement simmers down a bit and you're a little less sore, you'll be ready for a nice easy workout.

My recovery time was different with each child, and yours will be unique for you as well. For instance, any tearing will affect how you feel about exercising. But if you have an uncomplicated vaginal delivery, you can do some light exercises within the next few

AFTER-DELIVERY CHECKUP WITH DR. HELLER

How soon you can return to exercise depends on many factors. Most obvious, of course, is the route of delivery. If you had a C-section, your physician will be concerned about possible separation of the incision or hernia. It takes about six weeks for the abdominal fascia to return to 90 percent strength after any abdominal surgery. That means six weeks of no heavy lifting or straining after a C-section—any of these could increase the risk of hernia after surgery.

Even after a vaginal delivery, start back gradually. Most women can start with some light physical activity within a week. Remember, the uterus is still enlarged for six weeks: a weighted structure in the pelvic region, surrounded by connective tissue and muscle that has been stretched and stressed. Straining, heavy lifting, or sit-ups can cause the uterus or bladder to slip out of proper position, a condition known as pelvic prolapse. Basically, anything that increases abdominal pressure can strain the pelvic floor and make prolapse of the uterus or bladder more likely. Susceptibility to this is genetic to some degree—it depends on your collagen makeup—but any increased strain or lifting could make it more difficult for the anatomy to return to its original state.

Still, many women feel good, and I suspect that most women who return to exercise early don't ask their doctors about it. Most of them are going to be fine listening to their body. But if you are leaking urine, that's a sign that things are not back to normal. If you are aware of a bulge when you are urinating, if things don't feel toned or "the same" in the vaginal or vulvar area, or if you had stitches and you are still having pain, those are reasons for caution. Be conservative; do your Kegels.

days. Even if you feel fatigued, you'll probably at least want to take a walk in the first few days, then try some light upper-body moves. Of course, if you have a C-section, you have the whole surgical recovery to deal with, over and above recovering from delivery. See Dr. Heller's notes (above) and follow your medical team's advice to ensure a smooth and safe return to full activity.

No way around it, you will face some challenges in the early days postdelivery. Your pelvis will be sore—like a boxing title bout took place in your abdomen. Your abdominal muscles and skin are stretched out, and your uterus is still enlarged. Your weakened abs and the weight of the uterus may give you a backache, but this will not even compare to the back discomfort you experienced during the last month of pregnancy.

Your joints will still be a bit wobbly, too, from the lingering presence of relaxin. If you are a runner, your hips might be a bit unstable. No matter what your sport, your balance may not be back to what it once was. Stay on two feet for the first month or so at least, and only gradually introduce single-leg or other less stable exercises as your comfort level increases. Such things as bench dips, front squats, overhead presses, and crab walks may take a toll on the wrists, but stick with them for now, and trust me, you will get your balance back in a few weeks.

A challenge that may surprise you is how "down" you feel, especially when you think this ought to be the happiest moment of your life. This feeling is so common that there's a name for it: the "baby blues." It's totally normal to feel teary and unhappy for a week or so. You may feel isolated and burdened by your own expectations to be the perfect mom. Most women feel better after about ten days. If you are feeling low, don't pressure yourself by turning working out into yet another impossible to-do item on your list, just put the baby in a pack and get outside for a brisk walk. If it's pouring rain, turn on some great music and stomp around the house. Get moving. Exercise is one of the most time-honored treatments for depression of all kinds. If you don't feel better within a few weeks, bring it up at your postnatal visit.

BLEEDING

You leave the hospital with this amazing gauze underwear and a pad the size of a dictionary, but you will need these things so don't feel bad about sneaking some extras

> "After we'd been home 2 or 3 days I felt fine and I happily would have swam, but you have to stop bleeding first, so I started walking/jogging after about a week or two, just to get out—being cooped up is not my thing. When he was 5 weeks old I swam—the day after I stopped bleeding I went to the pool! But even though I can swim now, I've been running more because it's so convenient. You can leave the house and run for a half hour and get home afterward. It's nothing like driving to the pool, swimming, showering. That takes three hours."
>
> —KATE, SWIMMER, MOTHER OF ONE

into your bag to take home. The bleeding can be pretty heavy for about a week before it tapers off. This is totally normal as your body gets rid of the extra blood it manufactured early in the pregnancy to support the baby's growth. Once my bleeding slowed down, I started to exercise lightly, increasing the intensity as the bleeding lessened. Just be smart: if the bleeding is worse after your workout, then chill out for a day before you exercise again or drop back on the intensity. That is how I did it and that worked great. Use heavy pads (no tampons) and save your favorite workout clothes for later—you probably don't fit into them yet, anyway. As long as the bleeding is not excessive (passing clots or changing your pad every hour or two), it shouldn't interfere with your return to moderate exercise. And bear in mind that if you had an episiotomy or a tear it will take longer to heal and stop bleeding. Sit on an ice pack. Take warm baths. Do your Kegels to increase blood flow. This, too, will pass.

On the plus side, your heart rate will be back to normal, although you are probably so used to gauging your effort by the RPE scale that you may never return to your heart rate monitor.

I got back to a workout routine pretty quickly. I was very sore for about three days after Mackenzie, but felt better within the week. This allowed Steve and me to take her to the beach for a walk and some easy boot camp–style workout circuits, easing into it with brief upper- and lower-body exercises. After that I started to add strength training, doing more each week for about four weeks. For cardio, I concentrated on the recumbent bike (no way was I going to sit on my race bike seat after all that!), rowing machine, or walking for the first few weeks to let everything heal. But again, every pregnancy and delivery is different—just remember to trust your body and listen to yourself. You may not be getting back to exercise as quickly as you would like or expect, but keep in mind that there's no rush to a finish line. What's most important is that you take care of yourself and heal first.

Recent research indicates that some women are more fit *after* delivery than they were before the pregnancy! The body makes many adaptations to meet the demands of pregnancy—including improving oxygen uptake and pain tolerance. Many athletes who train through pregnancy show improved times and results in the aftermath. There is also evidence that the healing hormones your body produces postdelivery will give you an increased work capacity. Some women have seen significant increases their VO2Max and workload capacity.

This was quite evident with Brandi. Her power meter profile (biking power) was greater after a few weeks of bike training than it was before she became pregnant with our second child. There's no way to know if this was due to the training she went through during her pregnancy, or the hormonal bump she got as a result of being pregnant. Either way, she was stronger after giving birth to Maddox than she was before she got pregnant.

In a word, after delivery is a great time to increase your fitness, so don't let this opportunity pass you by. If you were fit going into the delivery, you will be able to get back to training quickly and use those "healing" hormones and additional blood volume to increase your overall fitness. Think of them as legal performance enhancement. As you rebuild your cardio capacity in the months following delivery, watch for this welcome boost.

Steve

"Coming back from my second, every distance race has been the fastest I've ever done. So I definitely feel I maintained my fitness, and having had the experience of having terrible runs for five, six, seven months—every run is better! I've heard that some women come back stronger runners. I used to be miserable on a 5K race—I don't feel that anymore and I'm faster than I ever was. It's been sixteen months—maybe I just got used to going faster."

—MOLLY, RUNNER, MOTHER OF TWO

GO EASY ON THE ABS

Most women, even sedentary ones, experience some urinary leaking after delivery, triggered by coughing, laughing, sneezing, or sometimes even just moving. During pregnancy we blamed this on the baby's weight on the bladder; now it's caused by the weakness—make that exhaustion—of the pelvic floor. Some women never get rid of this problem but most of us will, through exercises and time.

Your abdomen and core are definitely areas where you should "go slow to go fast." I know the urge to get to work on that belly right away is pretty strong, especially when you can see and feel how loose it is, but you don't need me to tell you that your entire pelvic region has been stretched and turned every which way, so be patient. Giving your pelvic floor time to recover will help you avoid serious long-term problems, such as a prolapsed uterus or bladder and leaking

urine. Let your pelvic floor return to its former shape and tone, and chances are this little problem will clear up quickly and not bother you anymore.

That means avoid any exercises that strain the abdominals or the pelvic floor, including any core work and lifting heavy weights. Don't do any one-rep maxes for a month at least and, if you hold your breath during heavier lifts, such as squats and deadlifts (Valsalva technique, see page 90), avoid that technique during this time to let that pelvic floor recover. For the first couple of days after delivery, just concentrate on flattening your abdomen when you exhale. Your abs are stretched out from carrying the baby—sometimes to more than twice their normal length! You have to give them a chance to shorten up first, and abdominal breathing will retrain them. Some Kegel exercises (see page 89 for a refresher) will also help set matters right in your pelvic floor. Practice holding a pelvic tilt by lying on your back with bent knees and flattening your back against the floor. Then try to hold the same position while standing against a wall.

Once you can maintain a good pelvic tilt, you can progress to bridges and heel slides. Then you can move to a few static planks, gentle curl-ups, and leg raises. If you feel pain, give yourself another day or two.

Do not rush the abdominals. If you are leaking urine when you exercise, you are working too hard. Back off, especially any lifting or core work. Do some Kegels, light cardio, and upper body instead. And remember the linea alba, that band between the rectus muscles down the center of your abdomen? If yours separated, lay off all abdominal exercises until your medical team gives you the go-ahead. A good general rule after delivery is to treat your body as if you were eight or nine months pregnant until you feel more comfortable and your body begins to feel normal again. If you follow those workouts or suggestions, you'll be in a good place.

SURPRISE BENEFITS OF PREGNANCY

Once you get moving again more consistently, chances are you will feel great. For one thing, you will be about 20 pounds lighter! Having a baby will be the fastest 12 pounds you ever lose, and another 5 pounds of fluids will drop off the scale in a day or so. So once you get settled into your routine, you may feel like you are flying along—and you probably are! Not only does the 60 percent increase in blood volume that pregnancy triggers result in more oxygen going to your muscles, but the hormones of pregnancy also increase muscle strength. (This boost is so well documented that in the 1970s and '80s some Eastern European countries were suspected of taking unethical advantage of it in an "abortion doping" scandal.)

Pregnancy confers another benefit that is a little surprising. Norwegian marathoner Ingrid Kristiansen claimed that childbirth boosted her athletic results by raising her pain threshold. Greg Whyte, professor of applied sport and exercise science at Liverpool John Moores University, puts it this way, "Women re-evaluate where they can anchor pain and many psychologists believe that woman's pain threshold is effectively reset so that when she resumes or takes up training again, nothing ever seems as uncomfortable." I experienced this with cycling. We go through a VO2Max step test to determine our max watts for the program. A couple of months after delivering Maddox, I joined the class and tested out at 290 watts. The following year I was about 30 watts less. Even through the entire program I could not get close to that 290 watts. I have determined that my pain tolerance was much higher and I could stay in the "pain cave" for much longer periods after my pregnancies.

GETTING BACK TO FIGHTING WEIGHT

I am sure most—if not all—competitive athletic women do not want to gain a lot of weight during their pregnancies because of the challenge of losing it postdelivery. This was one of my biggest concerns, too. Almost all women, athletes or not, ask how quickly they can lose all the baby weight. With Mackenzie I gained about 35 pounds. Although this may seem like a lot and it is more than many pregnant women gain, I took it in stride. I did not diet either time, just continued to eat the way I eat and move the way I move. Breast-feeding helped, too. It was amazing how the weight just melted off in a short period of time. Rest assured, you will lose yours, too, unless of course you do not get back on track with your fitness routine. In Dr. Clapp's studies, 55 percent of regular exercisers return to their prepregnancy weight and body fat ratio within six months, and 75 percent within one year. Several variables will affect how quickly you drop the pounds, including whether or not you opt for breast-feeding and how soon you get moving after delivery.

After the baby is born, give yourself a few weeks without dieting (which is a four-letter word, so only diet if you are not a healthy eater) to recover from labor and delivery—just as you would take some time off after an event. Then, if you are not breast-feeding, work your way back down to your prepregnancy calorie count. You can reduce calories if you want to speed weight loss, but not at the expense of nutrients. Whether or not you are breast-feeding, maintain a healthy and balanced diet. For nine months, the baby's needs have come first, and they still do if you are breast-feeding—the baby's nutritional needs will probably be met. Now is the time for your body to rebuild itself. Follow the same principles you followed while pregnant: plenty of nutrients, fiber, and vitamins and minerals—only now it's for you.

BREAST-FEEDING

Breast-feeding is a very personal choice, and so many factors play a role in it. Don't let anyone make you feel bad about not doing it if you can't or don't want to. I had hoped to breast-feed but I certainly underestimated how difficult it would be. Mackenzie had a little jaundice, enough for the doctor to recommend a couple nights' stay in the hospital under the blue lights. Of course I stayed in the hospital with her, giving me a few days of training with the nurses who will do anything to help you figure out how to breast-feed and connect with your baby with the "latching." Before this I was pretty shy and would never even change clothes in a public space. Suddenly I had three different women grabbing at and admiring my nipples! It took a while to really get it. I had my ups and downs and moments of wanting to give up, but there is something very magical about it that made me want to work hard and "get it" and hope the baby would get it too. Many women opt to breast-feed for the unique closeness with the baby and the extra health boost it offers to the newborn. It also has a reputation of making weight loss easier. I am sure I lost my baby weight much faster than if I had not breast-fed. The regimented schedule of feedings and pumping just doesn't work for everyone, but try to make it work even for the first three months.

Studies show that while many factors affect milk production, including your hormonal balance, nutrition, and whether you are pumping or nursing, exercise is probably not one of the important variables in milk supply. I lasted one year feeding Mackenzie until I dried up, barely able to pump a couple of ounces at the end. With Maddox the milk started to dwindle at six months. When you do stop breast-feeding, it is bittersweet.

I have never witnessed a greater athletic or physical challenge than natural childbirth—especially when it's the mother's first delivery. I have never met a woman as physically and mentally strong as Brandi, and to see her work as much and as hard as she did with the delivery of Mackenzie only strengthened my belief that women need to be as fit and healthy as possible when going into the delivery room so they can manage the delivery and recovery process. Granted, Brandi turned it into an "event" and set herself the challenge of getting Mackenzie out before Dido's shift ended at 7:00 p.m. (which she accomplished), but the effort she put in was Herculean. Delivering Maddox seemed much easier—at least it took a lot less time. But regardless of how long it takes, the event is incredibly taxing.

Steve

I breast-fed as long as I possibly could and really missed that connection with my babies when I stopped, but I admit that I totally loved having my body back to myself.

If you decide to breast-feed, be sure to increase your calories and hydration enough to support the baby in addition to any workouts and other activities you participate in (continuing to take in an extra 300 or so calories a day, as you did at the end of pregnancy, is a good place to start). Sleeping with a bra can help relieve the pressure in your breasts (you'll be carrying an extra 3 pounds of breast tissue!). Breast-feeding can be painful, somewhat inconvenient, and messy-bordering-on-gross (with milk leaking onto your bedsheets, bras, and clothes and everything smelling like spoiled milk). Still, some of the best memories you will have with your baby will be when you are breast-feeding him or her.

CAN YOU DIET WHILE YOU'RE NURSING?

Many women, athletes or not, look to breast-feeding as a time to lose any extra pounds they gained during pregnancy. As a new mother you can continue to exercise and even diet while you are breast-feeding, as long you consume enough calories to maintain the amount and quality of your milk. James Clapp's studies suggest that a caloric deficit of around 425 calories is the right balance. Keep your weight loss at ¾ to 1 pound a week—this is still three times faster than it would be if you just ate what you wanted, and it ensures enough milk for your baby's needs.

Be sure you eat enough: A tough workout can easily burn 600 calories. Breast-feeding takes calories, too—allot 300 a day early on and about 500 a day by the time the baby is a

---

TIP: FINDING TIME

How to get in a workout when you are on baby time? Here are some tips from new moms who have been there, done that:

- "Set up an old spin bike in the rec room and let the baby sleep in the corner."
- "You just have to tell yourself: 'It's happening. I am going to work out today.' Even though I was up all night, two weeks in, I was up at 4:30 feeding him and at the Y by 5:00."
- "It's really helpful to continue to do something so enjoyable. I'm home with the baby and not working right now but I still have two pool memberships. They have different open swim times and I work between them."
- "Have fun with it. If the weather is nice, load the baby up and head for the sidewalk. You can do walking lunges or butt kicks while you push. And the baby makes a handy 10-pound weight for shoulder presses, squats, lunges, or bridges!"

---

few months old. After all, you are feeding the baby from your body, just as you did during the pregnancy, and the baby is growing and needs more and more food. Continue grazing with complex carbs and enough protein and fats. Nutritionists say that nursing women need 20 grams more protein a day than they did before pregnancy—that's 10 grams a day more than during pregnancy. Be sure to take in enough calcium, because the baby's demands can leach calcium from your system (although your exercise program can help reduce bone loss). With these caveats in mind, follow the same dietary guidelines you adopted during pregnancy. Eat small, frequent meals of healthy foods and continue to avoid eating the big fish species (because of possible mercury contamination). Good news! You can have an occasional adult beverage! Just wait two hours between that glass

of wine and the next feeding (or pump and dump). Notice any foods that upset your baby's stomach (broccoli, garlic) or keep your child awake (caffeine, chocolate). Keep taking your vitamins (prenatal or regular), calcium, vitamin D, omega-3 supplements. Continue to eat wisely, so you and the baby make the most of your calories!

While it's natural to increase calories while you are breast-feeding, it's just as important to increase your fluids. Your body needs water to replace what it loses during exercise and to make milk. Your baby consumes 10 to 15 ounces of fluid daily at birth, and that amount increases every day! Remember to adjust your fluid intake accordingly. To avoid fatigue while exercising and to ensure your baby has enough milk, increase your water intake until your urine is pale yellow.

FINDING THE TIME

The first thing you learn as a new mom is that your time is not your own. Most athletes are pretty organized—we have to be to fit our workouts in between work, family life, and friends. You probably have your favorite time to hit the gym, the track, or the pool. You can probably kiss that favorite time good bye unless you have a great support system like your parents. A common scenario is you get yourself all ready to go to the gym, and then the baby's asleep. Or your gym offers daycare, but not until the baby is six weeks old. Or, at last the baby is asleep, but you can't go out for a run because you have to pump your milk. Now is when you will be glad you prepared for this a few months ago!

First, embrace flexibility. Once you start working out, accept that you may not be able to find an hour all at once, so break up your workout into short segments. When the weather's fine, load the baby into the stroller. Hit the gym at 5:00 a.m. before your partner goes to work. And remember that many of the workouts in this book are designed so you can do them at home with a minimal setup. Sure, you'll be tired, and most books tell you not to wear yourself out and sleep when the baby sleeps. But working out, even for 10 or 15 minutes a day in the beginning, will help you feel like yourself again, get those endorphins going again, and will help in your recovery (as long as you are taking these exercise sessions easy). The feeling of normalcy will be important: for a

> "Am I planning another? Absolutely! Based on how the first one went, I'd do it again. Working out did make it easier to get back into shape."
>
> —SUSAN, CYCLIST, MOTHER OF ONE

first-time parent, there is potentially nothing "normal" for you about having a baby in the house that requires 24-hour care! Find a way to fit it in. Like they say, "Just do it." Steve and I are very fortunate to have my mother to help with the kids when we need her. Being a mom, running a few businesses, and training to compete takes a lot of balance. My mom has truly helped us maintain our work and training schedules as the babies got older and I was not breast-feeding.

The fact is, everything will take longer once the baby is born. The logistics of breast-feeding add another dimension. But if you think you don't have time to breast-feed, consider for a moment the case of pentathlete (shooting, swimming, fencing, riding, running) Mickey Kelley, who returned to competition four months after delivery at age thirty-four. Kelley breast-fed her daughter between the fencing and swimming events at the 2012 World Cup. So if you do choose to breast-feed, rest assured that it *can* be done!

As you start on the road back to and beyond your prepregnancy peak, make your workouts progressively more challenging, taking into account the special modifications for the immediate postpartum period.

Start off gentle and move at your own pace. Base your pace and intensity on your blood flow. After four or five weeks I added more boot camp, run, bike, and swim workouts each week, until I was back to my full routine within six weeks. The volume was not where it was prepregnancy because I was not focused on any long events after either pregnancy, mostly sprint and Olympic distance for triathlon and 10K, with less running or adventure racing.

Don't rush it. As hard as this is to hear and even for me to say, what seems like forever when you are coming back is not a lot of time in the big picture of life. Listen to your body and take your time. It may be a cliché, but you will never have this time with the baby again so there's no reason to force yourself to work out when it's not enjoyable. Turn your workouts into nice breaks and "mommy time." Although it may seem to take forever, as it did for me, you'll be as good as new before you know it. Maybe even stronger and leaner!

If you don't want to get pregnant right away again, you might want to make sure you know the truth about pregnancy and breast-feeding—there's a pervasive myth that you can't get pregnant while breast-feeding. This is *definitely* an old wives' tale! So be careful unless you are ready for another bun in the oven!

SAMPLE POSTPARTUM STRENGTH WORKOUT

Modifications: The rowing machine (an ERG) and recumbent bike are very safe for the pelvic floor immediately postpartum. This makes them excellent postdelivery cardio exercises. Skip core and abdominal exercises for the first few weeks, focusing instead on the upper body. Save any jumping or high-impact aerobics until two months have passed.

Pay attention to your posture, and don't hunch over to push the stroller. Be sure to pump or nurse right before you run to reduce the pressure of your full boobs. Wear a comfortable and supportive nursing bra, with nursing pads to absorb any leaks. And remember to hydrate! Take water along for every workout.

The month after delivery will vary for each woman and every delivery. The best advice I can give is: don't obsess about working out. Focus on the baby's needs and your recovery. If you both are home from the hospital and everything is going well, you can start to think about getting moving. Keep it low intensity until you stop bleeding. Here are a couple workouts that I did in the first month after each pregnancy.

The Workouts

POSTDELIVERY WORKOUT 1

Equipment needed: Tubing (outdoor season)

Warm-up: Brisk walk pushing baby stroller (1–2 miles)

Conditioning: NONE!

Strength Circuit (6 exercises): Complete this circuit 3 times

Exercise #1: Air Squat (Squat focus)
Reps: 15

Exercise #2: Dumbbell (or Tubing) Chest Press (Push focus)
Reps: 20

Exercise #3: Dumbbell (or Tubing) Chest Fly (Push focus)
Reps: 20

Exercise #4: Tubing Back Row (Pull focus)
Reps: 20

Exercise #5: Bent Over, Straight-arm Tubing Pullbacks (Pull focus)
Reps: 20

Exercise #6: Bird Dogs (Core focus)
Reps: 10 per side

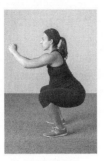

AIR SQUAT

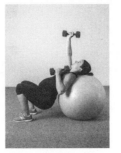

DUMBBELL (OR
TUBING) CHEST PRESS

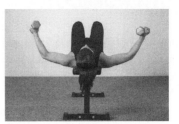

DUMBBELL (OR TUBING)
CHEST FLY

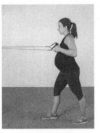

TUBING
BACK ROW

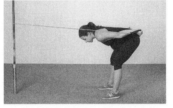

BENT OVER, STRAIGHT-ARM
TUBING PULLBACKS

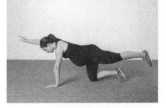

BIRD DOGS

Conditioning: Walk with stroller (1–2 miles)

Cool Down and Stretch:
   Static stretch, mobility work, foam roller: Follow the Stretch Routine introduced on page 18.

POSTDELIVERY WORKOUT 2 (3–4 WEEKS POSTDELIVERY)

Equipment needed: Cardio machine, physioball; dumbbells; agility ladder (indoor season)

Warm-up: Recumbent bike or treadmill walk (15–20 minutes)

Conditioning: Ladder Drills (6–8 rounds of any foot strike pattern of your choosing)

Strength Circuit (6 exercises): Complete this circuit 3 times

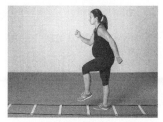

LADDER DRILLS

Exercise #1: Dumbbell Thruster (sit on the bench; tap your glutes to gauge your squat depth)

Reps: 15

Exercise #2: Dumbbell Physioball Chest Press (flat or incline) (Push focus)

Reps: 20

Exercise #3: Dumbbell Chest Fly (Push focus)

Reps: 20

Exercise #4: Single-arm Dumbbell Back Row (Pull focus)

Reps: 20

Exercise #5: Bent Over, Straight-arm Tubing Pullbacks (Pull focus)

Reps: 20

Exercise #6: Bird Dogs (Core focus)

Reps: 10 per side

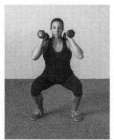

DUMBBELL THRUSTER

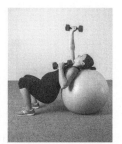

DUMBBELL PHYSIOBALL CHEST PRESS

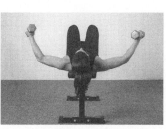

DUMBBELL CHEST FLY

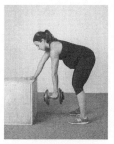

SINGLE-ARM DUMBBELL BACK ROW

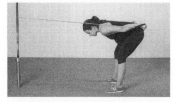

BENT OVER, STRAIGHT-ARM TUBING PULLBACKS

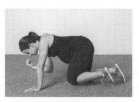

BIRD DOGS

Conditioning: Walk with stroller (1–2 miles)

Cool Down and Stretch:
Static stretch, mobility work, foam roller: Follow the Stretch Routine introduced on page 18.

Exercises

Here are the foundational movement categories we use to create workouts, along with some examples and possible modifications.

Type of Movement	Example Exercises	Modifications
Squat	Air Squat (Body Weight Squat), Back Squat, Front Squat, Split-Legged Squat, Sumo Squat	Can be done with barbell, dumbbells, kettlebells, resistance bands/tubing, and/or body weight. Increase the challenge by making the surface less stable or standing on one leg. Decrease the challenge by limiting the range of motion.
Push	Push-ups, Bench Press, Overhead Shoulder Press, Dips, Handstand Push-ups	Most exercises can be down with one or two arms. Can be done with barbell, dumbbells, kettlebells, resistance bands/tubing, and/or body weight.
Pull	Pull-ups, Ring Rows/Horizontal Pull-ups, Back Rows, Back Flies, Bicep Curls	Pull-ups can be made easier by using resistance bands.
Bend/Hip Flexion	Kettlebell Swings, Deadlifts, Romanian Deadlift (Double or Single Straight-Legged Deadlifts)	Most exercises can be done with barbell, dumbbells, kettlebells, resistance bands/tubing, and/or body weight.
Lunge	Front Lunges, Lateral Lunges, Reverse Lunges, Box Step-ups/downs, Pitcher Squats	Increase the challenge by incorporating resistance (plates, dumbbells, Kettlebells, medicine balls) and/or twisting.

continues

continued

Type of Movement	Example Exercises	Modifications
Conditioning/ Metabolic	Burpees, Mountain Climbers, Squat Jumps, ERG/Rowing	You will control the level of challenge, speed, and intensity at which you choose to do these exercises and movements.
Run/Plyometrics	Box Jumps, Broad Jumps, Sprinting, Jogging, Walking	You will control the level of challenge, speed, and intensity at which you choose to do these exercises and movements.
Compound Movements	Power Clean, Squat Clean, Clean and Jerk, Snatch, Thruster	Most can be done with barbell, dumbbells, or kettlebells.

General Pregnancy Precautions: As ligaments begin to loosen, be aware of your range of motion, not going too deep or too far away from the center of your body, and staying on both feet for heavier loads/weights.

Bend/Hip Flexion Focus

Ankle Band Air Squats (Bend/Hip Flexion and Squat focus)
1. Place an ankle band around both your ankles.
2. Stand with your feet shoulder-width apart and pull up ankle band around both legs to just below your kneecaps.
3. Perform a full-depth squat.
4. Repeat.

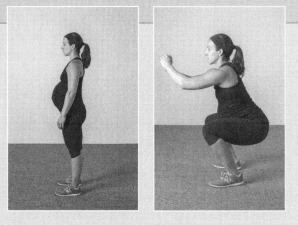

Barbell Romanian Deadlift (Bend/Hip flexion focus)
1. Stand with a shoulder-width or narrower stance. Grasp a barbell from the rack or deadlift from the floor with a shoulder-width or slightly wider overhand grip.
2. Lower the bar to the top of your feet by bending forward from your hips. Bend your knees during descent and keep your back straight so your back is parallel to the floor at the lowest position.
3. Lift the bar by extending at your hips and knees until standing upright. Pull your shoulders back slightly if rounded.
4. Repeat.

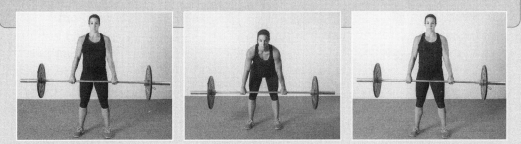

Bend/Hip Flexion Focus

Deadlifts (using a dumbbell or barbell) (Bend/Hip Flexion focus)

1. Stand with a shoulder-width or narrower stance with your feet flat beneath the bar. Squat down and grasp the bar with a shoulder-width or slightly wider overhand or mixed grip.

2. Lift the bar by extending your hips and knees to full extension. Pull your shoulders back at the top of the lift if rounded.

3. Return by bending your knees forward slightly while allowing your hips to bend back behind, keeping your back straight and knees pointed in the same direction as your feet.

4. Repeat.

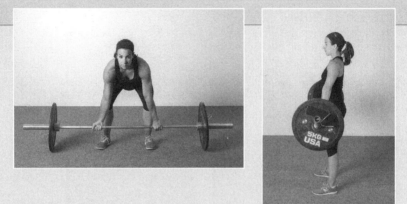

Dumbbell Romanian Deadlift/Straight-legged Deadlift (Bend/Hip Flexion focus)

1. Stand with your feet at shoulder width or narrower.

2. Grasp dumbbells to your sides.

3. With your knees straight, lower the dumbbells to top or sides of your feet by bending your hips.

4. Lift the dumbbells by extending your hips and waist until standing upright.

5. Pull your shoulders back slightly if rounded.

6. Repeat.

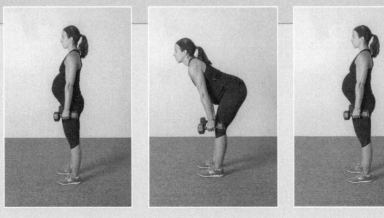

Bend/Hip Flexion Focus

Single-leg Romanian Deadlift (Bend/Hip Flexion focus)

1. Stand with a shoulder-width or narrower stance, holding a dumbbell in one hand.

2. Lower the dumbbell toward the ground, keeping your opposite leg on the ground and letting the leg on same side as the dumbbell rise off the ground behind you.

3. Bend your knees during descent and keep your back straight so your back is parallel to the floor at the lowest position.

4. Lift the dumbbell by extending at your hips and knees until standing upright. Pull your shoulders back slightly if rounded.

5. Repeat.

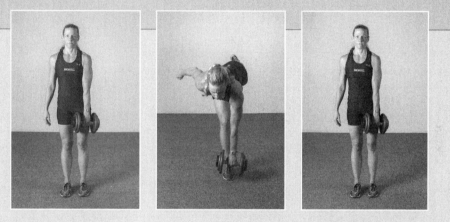

Snatch-grip Barbell Deadlift (Bend/Hip Flexion focus)

1. With your feet flat beneath the bar, squat down and grasp the bar with a snatch-width grip (hands out as wide as they can go) with an overhand or mixed grip.

2. Lift the bar by extending your hips and knees to a full extension. Pull your shoulders back at the top of the lift if rounded.

3. Return by bending your knees forward slightly while allowing your hips to bend back behind, keeping your back straight and knees pointed the same direction as your feet.

4. Repeat.

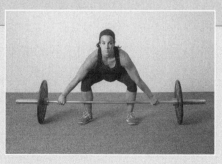 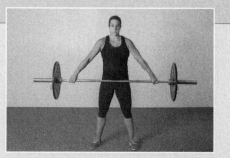

Compound Movements

Barbell Hang Clean (Compound Movement)

1. Stand holding a barbell with an overhand grip slightly wider than shoulder width. Feet point forward, hip width or slightly wider apart.

2. Bend your knees and hips so the barbell touches you at midthigh, keeping your shoulders over the bar with your back arched. Your arms are straight with their elbows pointed along the bar. Your chest is spread and your wrists are slightly flexed.

3. Jump upward, extending your body. Shrug your shoulders and pull the barbell upward with your arms, allowing your elbows to flex out to your sides, keeping the bar close to your body.

4. Aggressively pull your body under the bar, rotating your elbows around the bar. Catch the bar on your shoulders while moving into a squat position.

5. Hitting the bottom of the squat, stand up immediately. Bend your knees slightly and lower the barbell to the midthigh position.

6. Repeat.

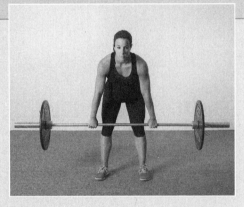
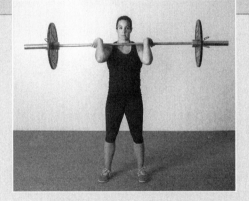

Barbell Push Jerk (Compound Movement and Push focus)

1. Stand holding the barbell with an overhand grip slightly wider than shoulder width.

2. Inhale and position your chest high with your torso tight. Keeping the pressure on your heels, dip your body by bending your knees and ankles slightly.

3. Explosively drive upward with your legs, driving the barbell up off your shoulders. Drop your body downward and split one foot forward and other backward as fast as possible while vigorously extending your arms overhead. The split position places your front shin vertical to the floor with your front foot flat on the floor. Your rear knee is slightly bent with your rear foot positioned on your toes. The bar should be positioned directly above your head at arms' length in line with your ears with your back straight.

4. Push up with both your legs. Position your feet side by side by bringing your front foot back partway and then your rear foot forward.

5. Lower the barbell to your shoulders. Then bend your knees slightly and lower the barbell to the midthigh position. Slowly lower the bar with a taut lower back and your trunk close to vertical.

6. Repeat.

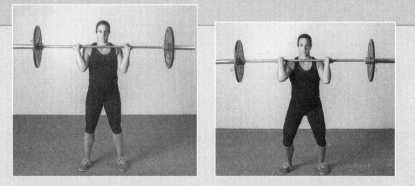

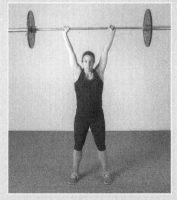

Note: The advanced athlete may unload (drop) the bar from the completed position. This technique may be practiced to reduce stress or fatigue involved in lowering the bar as prescribed. Use rubber weightlifting plates on a weightlifting platform if this unloading method is used (unless a floor demolition is desired).

Compound Movements

Burpee (Compound Movement)

1. Bend over and squat down. Place hands on the floor, slightly more than shoulder width apart.

2. Holding your upper body in place, kick your legs back. Land on your forefeet with your body in a straight plank position.

3. Perform a push-up by lowering your body to the floor and back up.

4. After your push-up, jump your feet as close to your hands as you can, preferably just outside your hands.

5. Explode up into a jump, reaching your hands over your head and clapping them together. Land with a soft bend in your knees.

6. Repeat.

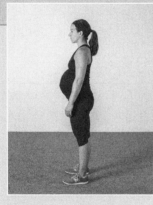

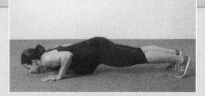

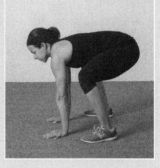

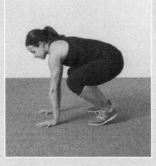

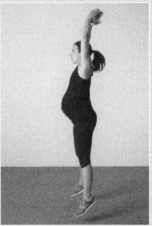

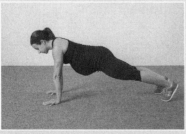

Compound Movements

Burpee or Squat Thrust–Broad Jumps (Compound Movement and Plyometrics)
1. Drop down into a push-up position; perform a push-up.
2. After your push-up, jump your feet as close to your hands as you can, preferably just outside your hands.
3. Explode up into a jump, reaching your hands over your head and clapping them together. Land with a soft bend in your knees.
4. Perform a forward broad jump, land, and drop back down into a push-up position.
5. Repeat.

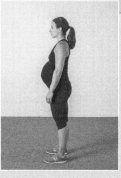
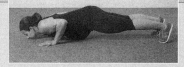
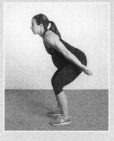
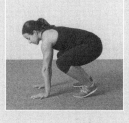
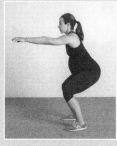
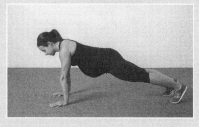
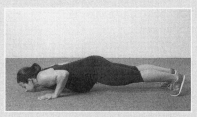
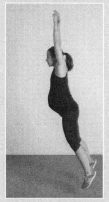

Compound Movements

Kettlebell Snatch (Compound Movement)

1. Straddle a kettlebell with your feet slightly more than shoulder width apart. Squat down with one arm extended downward between your legs and grasp the kettlebell handle with an overhand grip. Position your shoulder over the kettlebell with a taut low back and your trunk close to vertical.

2. Pull the kettlebell up off the floor by extending your hips and knees. Once the kettlebell is off the ground, vigorously raise your shoulder above the kettlebell while keeping the kettlebell between your knees.

3. Jump upward, extending your body. Elevate your shoulder and pull the kettlebell upward and forward. Aggressively pull your body under the kettlebell.

4. Catch the kettlebell at arm's length while moving into a squat position.

5. As soon as the kettlebell is caught on your locked-out arm in the squat position, stand with the kettlebell overhead.

6. Lower the kettlebell to front of your shoulder by bending your arm to the side. Drop the kettlebell forward and swing the kettlebell downward while squatting down with a taut lower back and your trunk close to vertical.

7. Set the kettlebell on the floor between your feet and repeat.

8. Continue with the opposite arm.

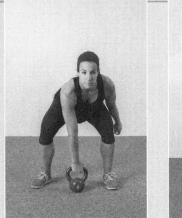
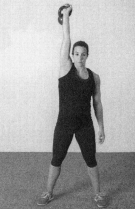

Kettlebell Sumo Squat High Pull (Compound Movement)
1. Stand over a kettlebell with a very wide stance.
2. Squat down and grasp the kettlebell handle with an overhand grip.
3. Lift the kettlebell by extending your hips and knees to their full extension.
4. Pull the kettlebell to chin height with your elbows leading—being pressed out to the sides.
5. Allow your wrists to flex as the kettlebell rises.
6. Lower and repeat.

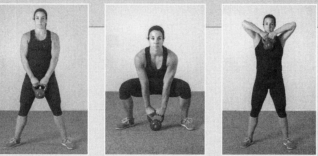

Kettlebell Swings (Compound Movement)
1. Straddle a kettlebell with your feet slightly more than shoulder width apart. Squat down with your arms extended downward between your legs and grasp the kettlebell handle with both hands with an overhand grip. Position your shoulder over the kettlebell with a taut low back and your trunk close to vertical.
2. Pull the kettlebell up and forward off the floor by standing up.
3. Immediately squat down slightly and swing the kettlebell back under your hips.
4. Quickly swing the kettlebell up by raising your upper body upright and extending your legs.
5. Continue to swing the kettlebell back down between your legs and up higher on each swing until its height just above your head can be maintained.
6. Swing the kettlebell back down between your legs. Allow it to swing forward but do not extend your hips and knees (as would be required to continue the swing).
7. Slow the kettlebell's swing and place on the floor between your feet in your original deadlift posture.
8. Repeat.

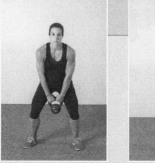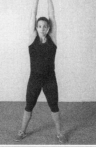

Compound Movements

Medicine Ball Squat Thrust, Throw, and Slam (Compound Movement)

1. Holding a medicine ball at waist level, drop down to a push-up position with your hands on the ball and your arms locked out.

2. Return to a standing position and throw the ball vertically 8 to 10 feet up so it touches/bounces off the wall and comes back down toward your hands.

3. Catch or let bounce, raise ball back over your head, and slam the ball to the ground, releasing the ball to let it bounce.

4. Catch the ball and repeat.

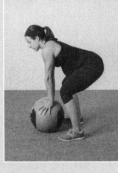
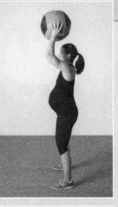
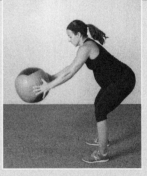

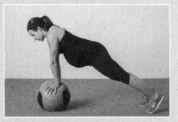
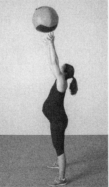
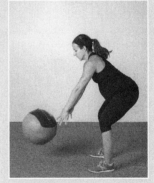

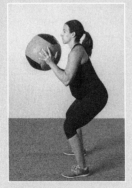
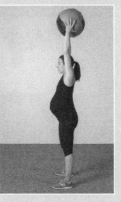

Medicine Ball Squat Thrust to Vertical Toss (Compound Movement)

1. Holding a medicine ball at waist level, drop down to a push-up position with your hands on the ball and your arms locked out.

2. Return to a standing position and throw the ball vertically 8 to 10 feet up so it touches/bounces off the wall and comes back down toward your hands.

3. Catch or let bounce and repeat.

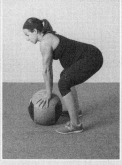

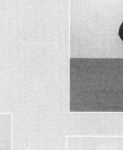

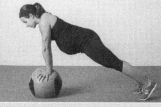

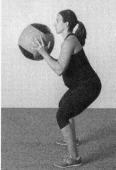

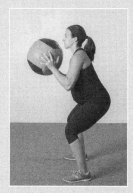

Compound Movements

Overhead Squat (Compound Movement)

1. Snatch or hang snatch a barbell overhead with a very wide overhand grip. Position your toes outward with a wide stance. Maintain the bar behind your head with your arms extended.

2. Descend until your knees and hips are fully bent or until your thighs are just past parallel to the floor. Your knees travel in the direction of your toes.

3. Extend your knees and hips until your legs are straight.

4. Return and repeat.

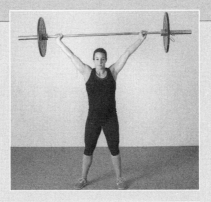

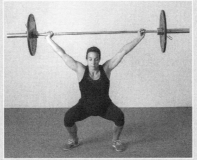

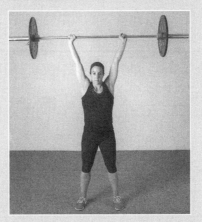

Push-Press (Compound Movement and Push focus)

1. Grasp a barbell from the rack or clean a barbell from floor with an overhand grip, slightly wider than shoulder width. Position the bar chest high with your torso tight. Retract your head back.

2. Dip your body by bending your knees, hips, and ankles slightly.

3. Explosively drive upward with your legs, driving the barbell up off your shoulders, vigorously extending your arms overhead.

4. Return the barbell to your shoulders and repeat.

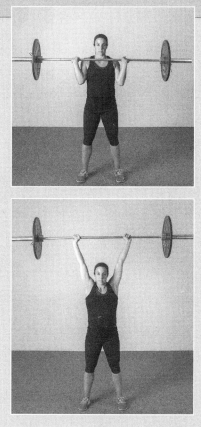

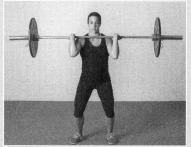

Compound Movements

Single-arm Dumbbell or Kettlebell Snatch (Compound Movement)

1. Stand with your feet apart and your toes pointing slightly outward.

2. Position a dumbbell or kettlebell in front of your thigh with your knuckles forward. Squat down with your back arched and lower the dumbbell between your knees with your arm straight and your shoulder over the dumbbell.

3. Pull the dumbbell up by extending your hips and knees. Jump upward, extending your body. Shrug your shoulders and pull the dumbbell upward with your arm, allowing your elbow to pull up to the side, keeping your elbow over the dumbbell for as long as possible.

4. Aggressively pull your body under the dumbbell. Catch the dumbbell at arm's length while moving into a squat position.

5. As soon as the dumbbell/kettlebell is caught on your locked-out arm in the squat position, move into a standing position with the dumbbell overhead.

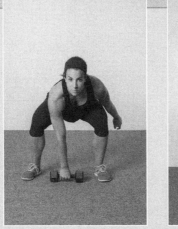
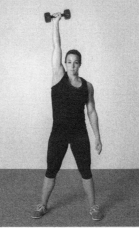

Compound Movements

Single-leg Medicine Ball Slams (Compound Movement)
1. Standing on one leg, raise a medicine ball above your head
2. Drive your arms down while throwing the ball to the floor and catch on its first bounce.

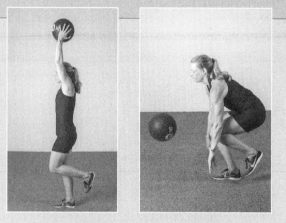

Kettlebell Sumo Squat High Pull (Compound Movement)
1. Stand over a kettlebell with a very wide stance.
2. Squat down and grasp the kettlebell handle with an overhand grip.
3. Lift the kettlebell by extending your hips and knees to their full extension.
4. Pull the kettlebell to chin height with your elbows leading—being pressed out to the sides.
5. Allow your wrists to flex as the kettlebell rises.
6. Lower and repeat.

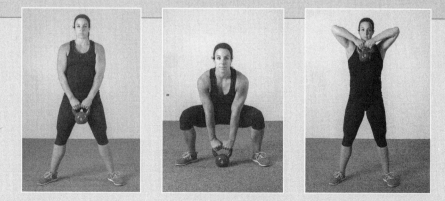

Compound Movements

Thruster (dumbbell or barbell) (Compound Movement)

1. From the floor (first repetition only) power clean a barbell up to your shoulders/front rack position.

2. Perform a front squat and when standing, press the barbell straight up until your arms are locked out overhead.

3. Pause, then lower the barbell back to the front rack position.

4. Perform a front squat, stand with an overhead press, then lower to the front rack position.

5. Repeat step 4.

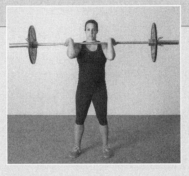

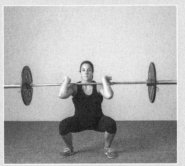

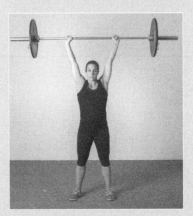

Tire Flip (Compound Movement)

1. Begin by going into a deep squat, gripping the bottom of a tire on the tread, and position your feet back a bit. Your chest should be driving into the tire.

2. To lift the tire, extend through your hips, knees, and ankles, driving into the tire and up.

3. As the tire reaches a 45-degree angle, step forward and drive a knee into the tire. As you step forward, adjust your grip to the upper portion of the tire and push it forward as hard as possible to complete the turn.

4. Repeat.

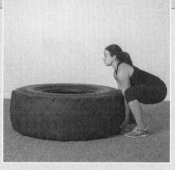
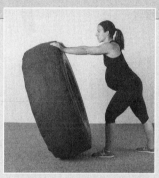
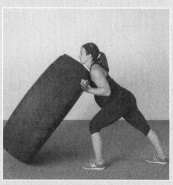
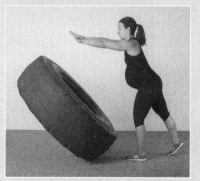

Compound Movements

Sledgehammer Tire Slam Tabata (Compound Movement and Metabolic focus)
4 minutes: 20 seconds hit tire, rest 10 seconds. Repeat for 8 rounds.

1. Stand facing a tire, about 2 feet away from it. If you are swinging from your right side, your left foot should be 3 to 5 inches closer to the tire than your right.

2. Grip the sledgehammer with your left hand at the bottom of the handle, and your right hand closer to the head.

3. Bring the hammer over high over your right shoulder, letting your right hand slide toward the head; as you swing down, slide your right hand down to join your left hand.

4. Slam the sledgehammer down as hard as you can against the tire, then control the bounce. Controlling the bounce is an integral part of the exercise, recruiting several stabilizer muscles, including those of your wrists and forearms.

5. Switch hands every few reps.

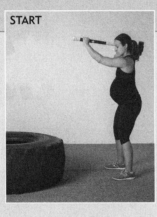

START

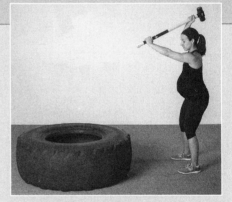

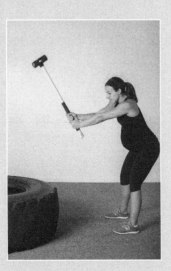

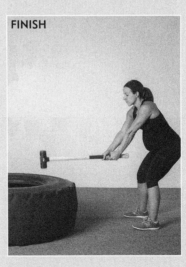

FINISH

Wood Chops (Compound Movement)

1. Holding a medicine ball, raise your arms centered above your head (with a slight bend in your elbows)

2. Bring the weight toward the floor, by dropping your arms and bringing the ball between your legs, squatting and flexing at the waist without letting the ball hit the floor.

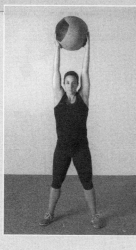
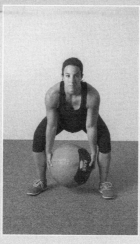
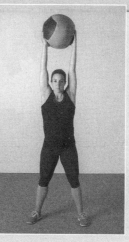

Conditioning/Metabolic Focus

(*Conditioning* and *metabolic* essentially mean the same thing, and you'll hear both terms, depending on the setting you where work out. At CrossFit facilities it's referred to as "metcon" (metabolic conditioning).

Barbell Burpee Jump-overs (Conditioning/Metabolic focus)
1. Stand facing or parallel to a barbell.
2. Complete 1 burpee, then jump over the barbell.
3. Turn around and complete the next burpee on the opposite side of the barbell.
4. Repeat.

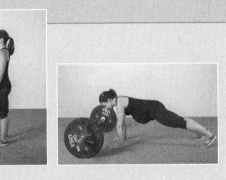 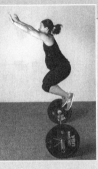 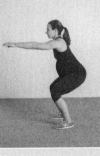

Double-unders (jump rope) (Conditioning focus)
1. Jump and swiftly swing the rope around your body and under your feet twice before landing.
2. Repeat.

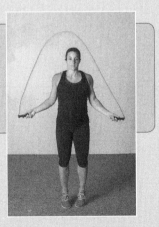

Dot Hops (Conditioning focus)

Move from one exercise to the next, resting only as much as you need to.

1. Double-legged plyo-hops forward and backward
2. Double-legged plyo-hops side to side
3. Single-leg (leg 1) plyo-hops forward and backward
4. Single-leg (leg 2) plyo-hops forward and backward
5. Single-leg (leg 1) plyo-hops side to side
6. Single-leg (leg 2) plyo-hops side to side

Reps: 30 seconds each

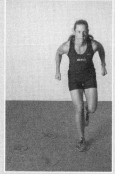
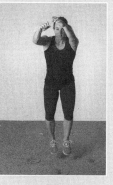
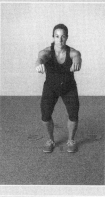
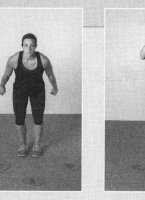
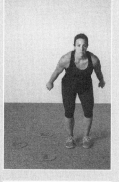
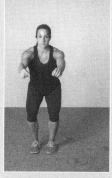
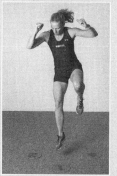
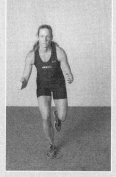

Conditioning/Metabolic Focus

Dumbbell Farmers Carry (Conditioning focus)

1. With a heavy dumbbell in each hand, walk the prescribed distance, trying not to put the weight down.

2. Turn around and return.

Reps: 50 yards

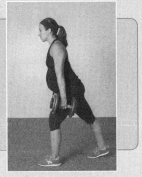

Dumbbell Thrusters (Conditioning focus)

1. Stand with the two dumbbells at shoulder height with a neutral grip (palms toward shoulders)

2. Perform a front squat and then stand, pressing the dumbbells straight up until your arms are locked out overhead.

3. Pause, then lower the dumbbells back to the side of your shoulders.

4. Repeat steps 2 and 3.

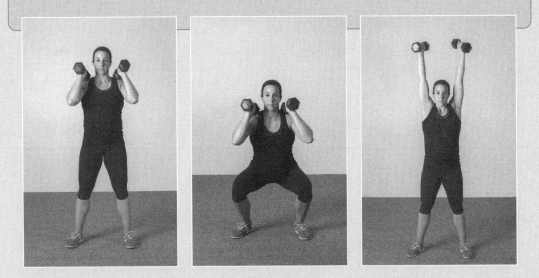

Conditioning/Metabolic Focus

Ladder Drills (Conditioning focus)
6–8 rounds of any foot strike pattern of your choosing

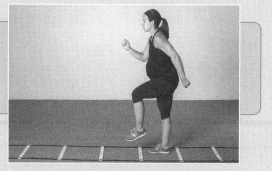

Shuttle Run (Conditioning focus)
Run out the prescribed distance, run back to start point, run back out the prescribed distance, and run back to start.

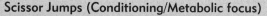

Scissor Jumps (Conditioning/Metabolic focus)
1. Stand with one foot forward and other foot back with your knees initially bent only slightly. Dip your body down by bending your legs more.
2. Immediately jump upward. Quickly reposition your legs and land with your feet in opposite positions.
3. Immediately dip your body down by bending your legs, with your rear knee almost making contact with the floor. Keep your torso upright and the hip of the rear leg straight.
4. Repeat the sequence with opposite leg movement. Continue the jumps while alternating your leg positions.

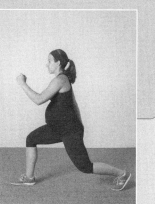

Conditioning/Metabolic Focus

Sledgehammer Tire Slam Tabata (Compound Movement and Metabolic focus)
4 minutes: 20 seconds hit tire, rest 10 seconds. Repeat for 8 rounds.

1. Stand facing a tire, about 2 feet away from it. If you are swinging from your right side, your left foot should be 3 to 5 inches closer to the tire than your right.

2. Grip the sledgehammer with your left hand at the bottom of the handle, and your right hand closer to the head.

3. Bring the hammer over high over your right shoulder, letting your right hand slide toward the head; as you swing down, slide your right hand down to join your left hand.

4. Slam the sledgehammer down as hard as you can against the tire, then control the bounce. Controlling the bounce is an integral part of the exercise, recruiting several stabilizer muscles, including those of your wrists and forearms.

5. Switch hands every few reps.

START

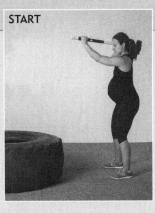
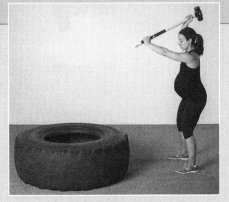

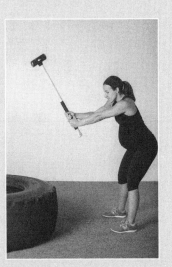
FINISH
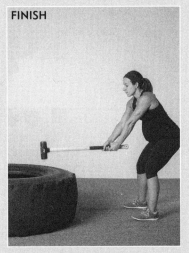

Weighted Drive Sled Push (Conditioning)

1. Stand facing a drive sled with your feet staggered. Bend down and grasp the handles or edge with both hands. Position your hips low, foot back, torso nearly horizontal, and arms straight.

2. On start, rapidly lean your body weight into the sled by dropping your body downward with your heels off the ground. Keep your weight low behind the sled while stepping forward as rapidly as possible.

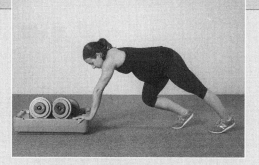

Conditioning/Metabolic Focus

Rowing (Conditioning focus)

1. Sit on the seat, strap your feet into the foot pads, and grab the handles with an overhand grip.

2. Extend your arms straight toward the flywheel, and keep your wrists flat.

3. Slide forward on the seat until your shins are vertical.

4. Lean forward slightly at the hips.

The Drive Position

1. Begin the drive by extending your legs and pushing off against the foot pads.

2. Keep your core tight, arms straight, and back firm as you transfer power to the handles.

3. As your knees straighten, gradually bend your arms and lean your upper body back. Finish with a slight backward lean.

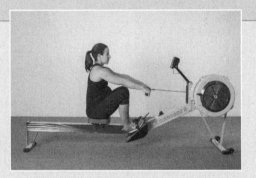
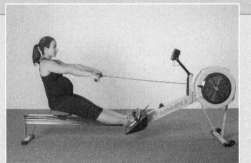

Rowing (Conditioning focus) *continued*

The Finish Position

1. Bend your elbows and pull the handle into your abdomen.
2. Extend your legs.
3. Lean back slightly at the hips.

The Recovery Position

1. Extend your arms by straightening your elbows and returning the handle toward the flywheel.
2. Lean your upper body forward at the hips to follow your arms.
3. Gradually bend your knees and slide forward on the seat to the start position.

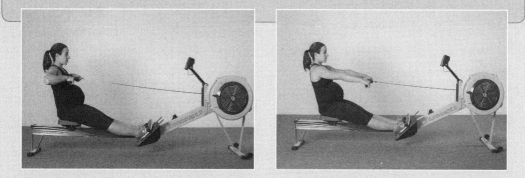

The Catch Position

1. Similar to the start position, extend your arms straight toward the flywheel and keep your wrists flat.
2. Slide forward on the seat until your shins are vertical.
3. Lean forward slightly at the hips.
4. You are ready to take the next stroke.

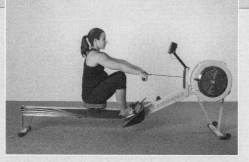

Core Focus

Ab Trilogy (Core focus)
1. With feet flat on the floor, crunch.
2. With your legs at 90-degree angle, crunch.
3. With your legs raised straight above your head, crunch.

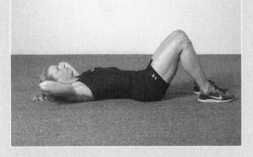
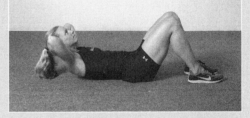
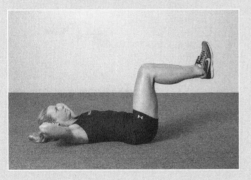
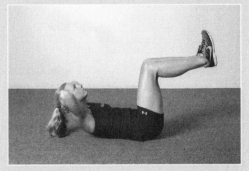
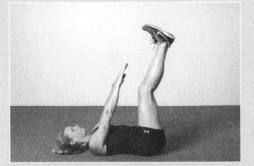
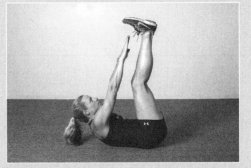

Bent Leg V-ups/Jack Knife (Core focus)
1. Sit on the floor or a mat.
2. Lie supine with your hands to your sides.
3. Simultaneously raise your knees and torso until your hips and knees are flexed.
4. Return to the starting position with your waist, hips, and knees extended.
5. Repeat.

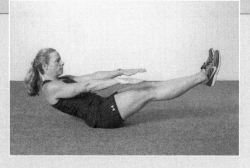 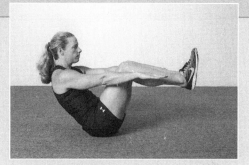

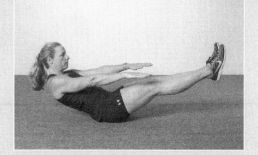

Core Focus

Bird Dogs (Core focus)
1. Kneel on a mat on all fours with your legs and hands slightly apart.
2. Raise one arm out straight beside your head while raising and extending the opposite leg behind your body.
3. Lower your arm and leg to the floor to their original position.
4. Perform the movement with your opposite arm and leg and repeat.

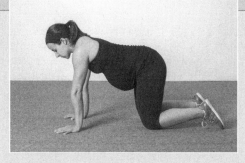
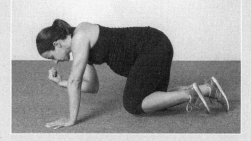
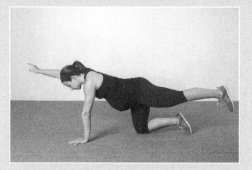

Core Focus

Diagonal Abdominal Suitcase (Core focus)
1. Sit on the floor or a mat.
2. Bend your knees, then crunch, bringing your knees closer to abdomen and twisting your torso from side to side.

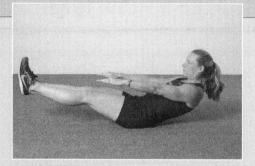
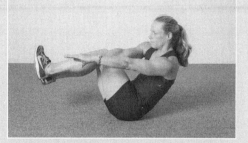

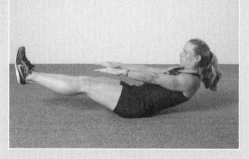

Core Focus

Dumbbell Plank Rows (Core and Pull focus)

1. Start in a plank position with a dumbbell in each hand.

2. Pull one dumbbell to your side until your upper arm is just beyond horizontal or the height of your back.

3. Return the dumbbell to the ground. Alternate your arms.

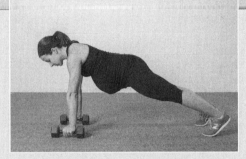 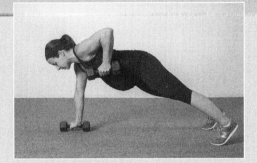

Forearm/Front Plank (Core focus)

1. Lie on your stomach with your elbows close to your sides and directly under your shoulders, palms down and fingers facing forward.

2. Slowly lift your torso and thighs off the floor. Keep your torso and legs rigid. Do not allow any sagging in your rib cage or low back. Hold this position.

3. Lower your body back toward the floor.

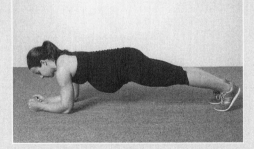

Core Focus

Inchworm Walkout (Push and Core focus)

1. From a standing position with your feet together or slightly apart, bend forward from your hips. Try to keep your legs straight (without locking your knees).

2. Put your hands on the ground and begin to walk your hands forward, away from your feet, until a full push-up position is reached.

3. Perform one full push-up.

4. Keeping your legs straight, walk your hands back to your feet.

5. Repeat.

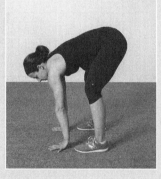

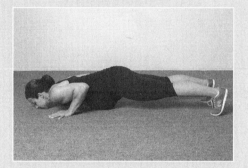

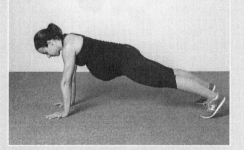

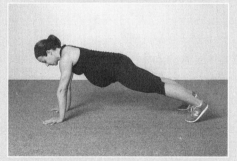

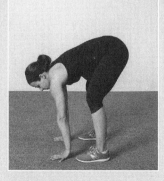

Core Focus

Medicine Ball Butterfly Sit-up (Core focus)

1. Lie on your back with your knees bent, the soles of your feet together, and a medicine ball above your head.

2. Sit up to touch the ball to your feet.

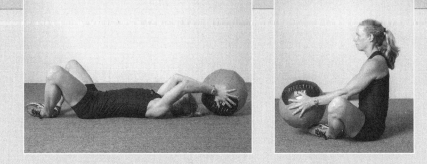

Medicine Ball Chattanooga Push-ups (Core and Push focus)

1. With a medicine ball under one hand, drop to a push-up while drawing your leg (medicine-ball side) out to the side of your body—pulling your knee up toward your elbow.

2. Switch the medicine ball and repeat on other side.

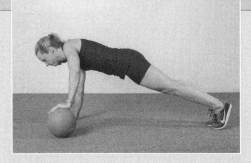 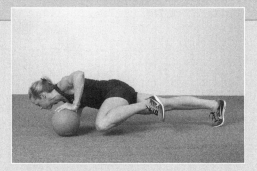

Core Focus

Medicine Ball Straight-legged Ab Pulses (Core focus)
1. Lie on your back with your feet in the air and your legs straight.
2. Hold a medicine ball in your hands, arms outstretched toward your feet.
3. Crunch up to touch your toes.

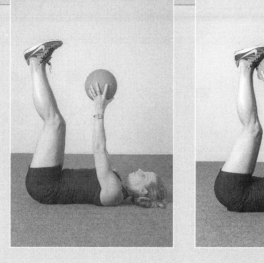

Physioball ABCs Plank (Core focus)
1. Start in a plank position on a physioball with your hands together.
2. By moving your forearms while on the ball, draw the shape of each letter of the alphabet. Try to make each letter 4 to 6 inches in size.

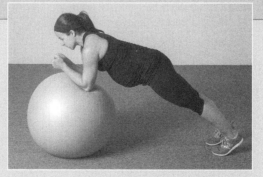

Core Focus

Physioball Transfer (Core focus)

1. Lying on your back, hold a physioball between your feet.

2. Raise your legs toward your head (V-up movement, keeping your arms and legs straight) carrying the ball in your feet.

3. Take the ball into your hands from your feet and lower the ball to the floor behind your head while returning your feet toward the ground.

4. Reverse the motion, bringing the ball back into your feet to complete the exercise.

5. Repeat.

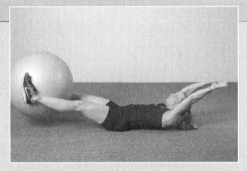 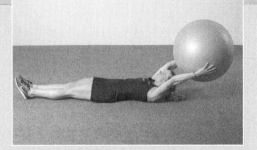

Physioball Walkout w/Push-up and Knee Tuck (Core and Push focus)

1. Start on your stomach on a physioball. Roll out forward so just your shins are on the ball.

2. Complete 1 push-up and then complete 1 knee tuck, pulling your thighs up into your chest.

3. Roll back until your chest is back on the ball.

4. Repeat.

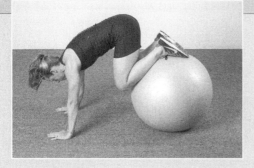 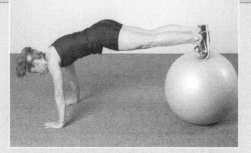

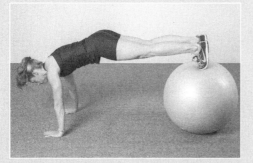 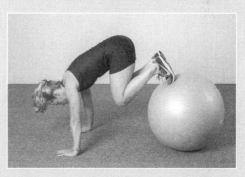

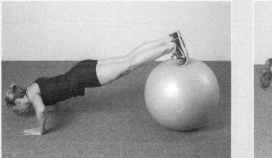 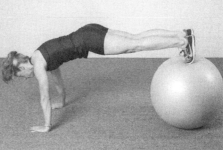

Core Focus

Side Bridge (Core focus)

1. Lie on your side on a mat. Place your bottom forearm on the mat under your shoulder perpendicular to your body. Place your upper leg directly on top of your lower leg and straighten your knees and hips.
2. Raise your hips upward by a lateral flexion of your spine.
3. Lower to your original position and repeat.
4. Repeat with the opposite side.

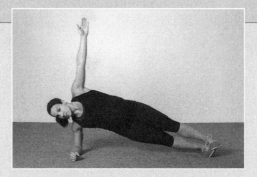

Superman Hold (Core focus)

1. Lie prone on a mat with your legs together and arms extended out on the floor, approximately parallel.
2. Slowly raise your upper body and legs off the floor and hold briefly.
3. Return your upper body and legs to the floor.
4. Repeat.

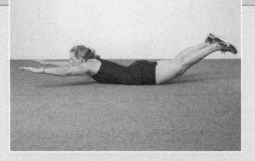

Superman Pulse-up (Core focus)

1. Lying on your stomach, raise your arms and legs at the same time, then lower to the ground in a fluid motion.

2. Repeat.

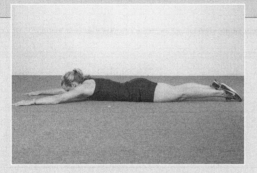 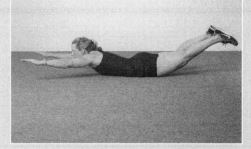

Core Focus

Yoga Push-up (Push and Core focus)

1. Start in pike/Downward Facing Dog position.

2. Leading with your head, bend your arms and lower your body in a scooping motion to the floor, finishing in a Cobra position. Your body never touches/rests on the floor.

3. Reverse the motion to complete the move.

4. Repeat.

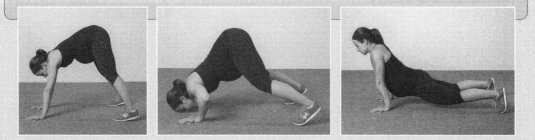

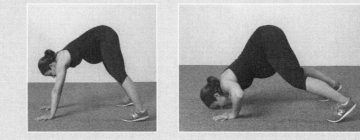

Lunge Focus

Ankle Band Lateral Shuffle (Lunge focus)
1. Stand with an ankle band around your ankles.
2. Side shuffle out and back, maintaining a three-quarter squat position.

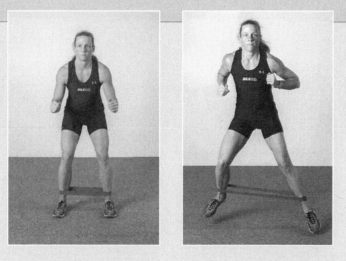

Bosu Lateral Lunge (Lunge focus)
1. Start beside a Bosu ball with your feet together on the ground.
2. Step one foot sideways onto the Bosu, ending in a lateral lunge position.
3. Press off the Bosu, returning to your beginning position.
4. Repeat. Complete all repetitions on the first side, then switch to the second side.

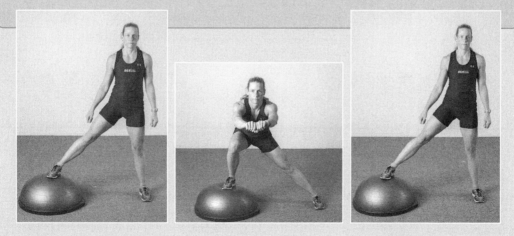

Lunge Focus

Step-up to Reverse Lunge (with or without dumbbell) (Lunge focus)
1. Step up to a full upright position on a box.
2. Drop your nonstanding leg back to the lunge position. Try to touch your back knee to the floor.
3. Return both feet to the floor.
4. Step up next with your back leg (you will alternate feet).

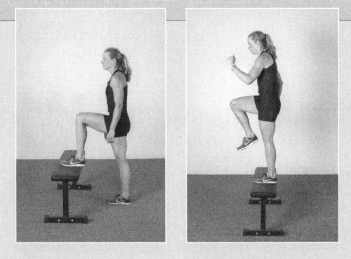

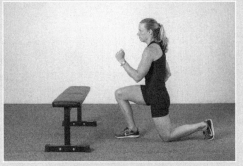

Note: If you are going to add weight, start light—5 to 8 pounds—and if you can still get through 3 sets of 20 reps without significant challenge, increase the weight. Choose a weight that creates challenge but as soon as your form and technique are compromised, decrease the weight.

Dumbbell Forward Lunge (Lunge focus)

1. Holding one or two dumbbells, step forward with your first leg. Land on your heel, then on your forefoot.

2. Lower your body by flexing your knee and hip of your front leg until the knee of your rear leg is almost in contact with the floor.

3. Stand up on your forward leg with the assistance of your rear leg.

4. Lunge forward with your opposite leg. Repeat by alternating the lunge with the opposite legs.

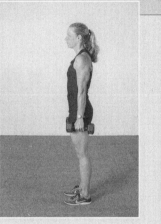 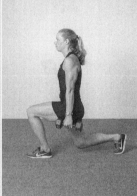

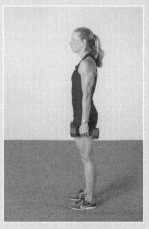

Lunge Focus

Forward Quarter Lunge (Lunge focus)
1. Perform a forward lunge, but only descend one-quarter of the way down.
2. Stand on your forward leg with the assistance of your rear leg.

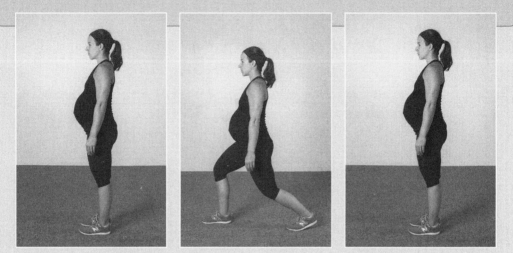

Lateral Lunge (with or without dumbbell) (Lunge focus)
1. Lunge to one side with your first leg, landing on your heel. then on your forefoot.
2. Lower your body by flexing the knee and hip of your lead leg, keeping the knee pointed in the same direction as your foot.
3. Return to your original standing position by forcibly extending the hip and knee of your lead leg.
4. Repeat by alternating the lunge with your opposite leg.

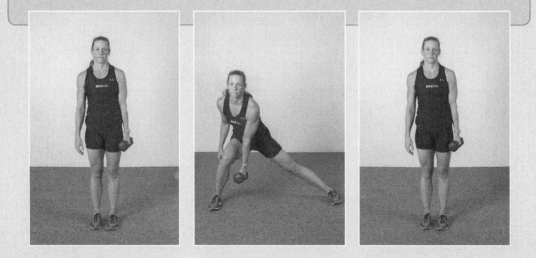

Lunge Focus

Overhead Plate Hold Forward Lunge Walk (Lunge focus)

1. Hold a weight plate overhead with locked-out arms.
2. Step forward with the first leg, landing on your heel, then on your forefoot. Lower your body by flexing the knee and hip of your front leg until the knee of your rear leg is almost in contact with the floor.
3. Stand on your forward leg with the assistance of your rear leg.
4. Lunge forward with opposite leg.
5. Repeat by lunging with alternating legs.

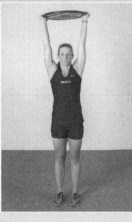 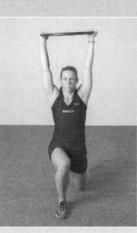 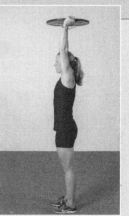

208

Metabolic/Conditioning Focus

10-9-8s (Metabolic/Conditioning focus)

Select one or two compound movement exercises and one sprint or other metabolic.
1. Perform each exercise 10 times.
2. Perform each exercise 9 times.
3. Perform each exercise 8 times.
4. And so forth, all the way down to 1.

Barbell Burpee Jump-overs (Metabolic/Conditioning focus)
1. Start facing or parallel to a barbell.
2. Complete 1 burpee, then jump over the barbell.
3. Turn around and complete the next burpee on the opposite side of the barbell.
4. Repeat.

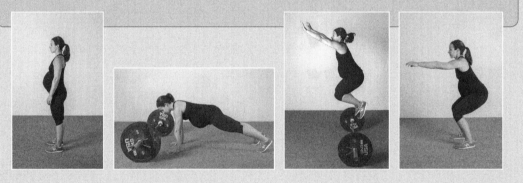

Mountain Climber (Metabolic focus)

1. Place your hands on the floor, slightly more than shoulder width apart. On your fore-feet, position one leg forward, bent under your body, and extend other leg back.

2. Hold your upper body in place and alternate your leg positions by pushing your hips up while immediately extending your forward leg back and pulling your rear leg forward under your body, landing on both forefeet simultaneously.

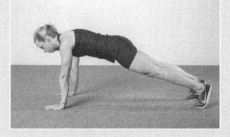
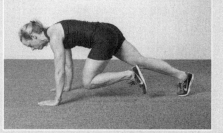

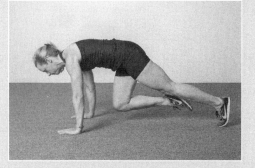

Metabolic/Conditioning Focus

Scissor jumps (Conditioning/Metabolic focus)

1. Stand with one foot forward and the other foot back with your knees initially bent only slightly. Dip your body down by bending your legs more.

2. Immediately jump upward. Quickly reposition your legs and land with your feet in the opposite positions.

3. Immediately dip your body down by bending your legs just short of your rear knee, making contact with the floor. Keep your torso upright and the hip of your rear leg straight.

4. Repeat the sequence with opposite leg movement. Continue the jumps while alternating leg positions.

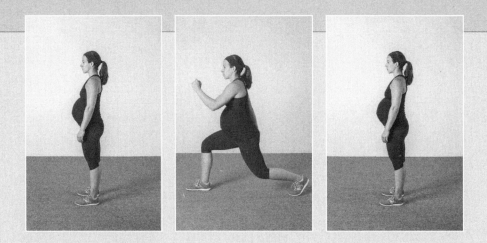

Tabata (Metabolic focus)

Select an exercise. Perform at high intensity for 20 seconds, followed by 10 seconds of rest. Repeat 8 times for a total training time of 4 minutes. You may alternate between two exercises if you wish.

Plyometrics

Box Jumps (Plyometric)
1. Stand in front of a secured box or platform.
2. Jump onto the box and immediately back down to the same position.
3. Immediately repeat.
Modify by stepping down and pausing between each jump and descent.

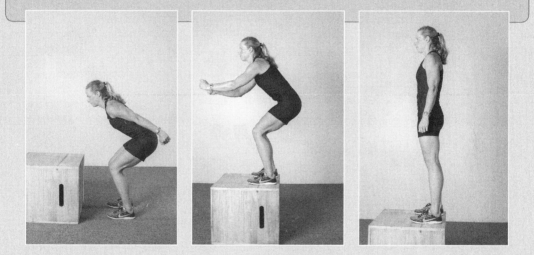

Plyometrics

Broad Jump (Plyometric)

1. Squat down and jump as far forward as possible, cushioning the landing with "soft" knees.

2. Upon landing, immediately jump out again.

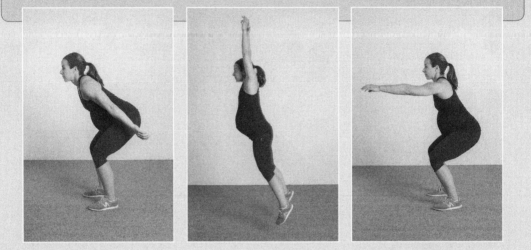

Squat Jumps (Plyometric)

1. Squat down and jump up as high as possible, cushioning the landing with "soft" knees.

2. Upon landing, immediately jump up again.

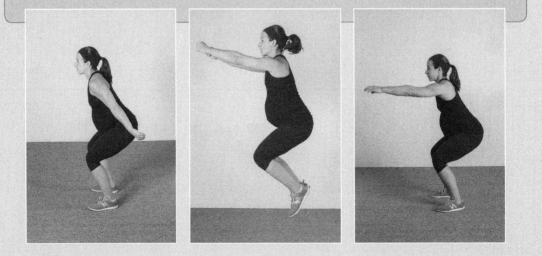

Pull Focus

Bent Over, Straight-arm Tubing Pullbacks (Pull focus)
1. Secure tubing on a support. Bend at your waist so your torso is roughly parallel to the ground.
2. Grab the tubing handles and pull the handles all the way back past your hips and return the handles back to the start position.
3. Repeat.

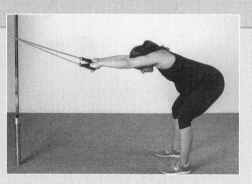 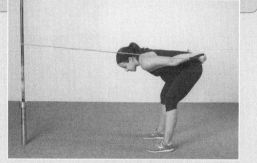

Dumbbell Plank Rows (Core and Pull focus)
1. Start in a plank position with one dumbbell in each hand.
2. Pull one dumbbell to your side until your upper arm is just beyond horizontal or the height of your back.
3. Return the dumbbell to the ground. Alternate your arms.

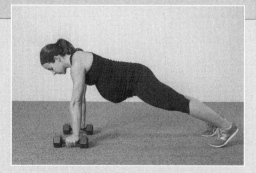 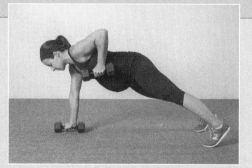

Pull Focus

Dumbbell Single-arm Bicep curl (Pull focus)

1. Hold two dumbbells at your sides, palms facing in, arms straight.

2. With your elbows to your sides, raise one dumbbell and rotate your forearm until your forearm is vertical and your palm faces your shoulder.

3. Lower to the original position and repeat with your opposite arm.

4. Continue to alternate between sides.

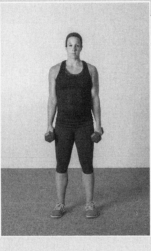 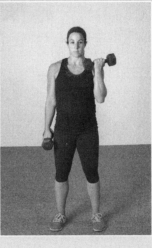

Dumbbell Single-arm Bicep Curl to Overhead Press (Push and Pull focus)

1. Position two dumbbells to your sides, palms facing in, arms straight.

2. With your elbows to your sides, raise one dumbbell and rotate your forearm until your forearm is vertical and your palm faces your shoulder.

3. With the dumbbell at shoulder level, press the weight straight up, finishing with your arm locked out and your bicep close to your ear.

4. Lower the weight back to your side and continue to alternate between sides.

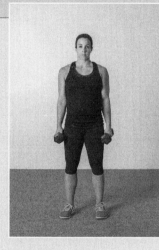 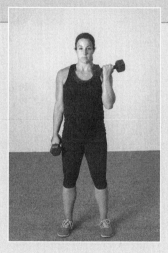 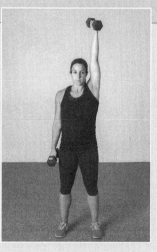

Pull Focus

Physioball Double-leg Hamstring Curls (Pull focus)

1. Lie supine on the floor with your lower legs on an exercise ball, your arms extended out to the side.

2. Straighten your lower back, knees, and hips, raising your back and hips off the floor.

3. Keeping your hips and lower back straight, bend your knees, pulling your heels toward your rear end. Allow your feet to roll up onto the ball.

4. Lower to your original position by straightening your knees.

5. Repeat.

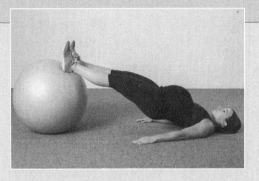
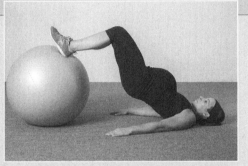

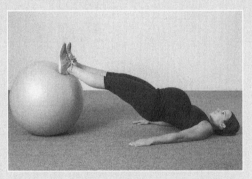

Pull Focus

Physioball Single-leg Hamstring Curls (Pull focus)

1. Lie supine on the floor with one lower leg on an exercise ball, the other leg in the air with knee bent, and your arms extended out to the side.

2. Straighten your lower back, knees, and hips, raising your back and hips off the floor.

3. Keeping your hips and lower back straight, bend the leg on the ball, pulling your heel toward your rear end. Allow your foot to roll up onto the ball.

4. Lower to your original position by straightening your knee.

5. Repeat.

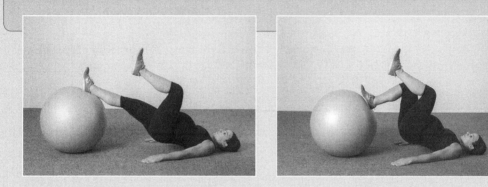

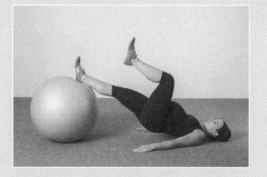

Pull Focus

Physioball Single-arm Row (Pull focus)
1. Stand with one hand on a physioball or bench and a dumbbell in the opposite hand.
2. Draw the dumbbell back to midchest level, then straighten your arm.
3. Repeat.

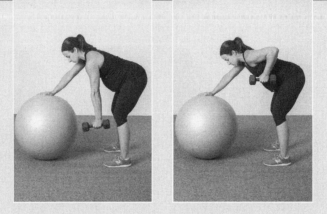

Plank Single-arm Dumbbell Reverse Fly (Pull focus)
1. Start in a plank/push-up position with a dumbbell in one or both hands.
2. Raise one arm out straight to the side (laterally).
3. Lower dumbbell back to the floor.
4. Alternate sides and repeat.

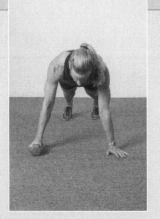
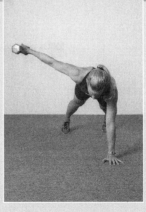

Pull Focus

Pull-up (Pull focus)

1. Begin with an overhand grip on the bar, palms facing away from you
2. Pull your body up until your chin is above the bar.
3. Lower your body until your arms and shoulders are fully extended.
4. Repeat.

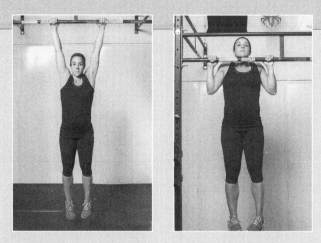

Ring/TRX Rows (Pull focus)

1. With your arms slightly bent and holding a handle in each hand, lean back to add tension to the straps. Walk your feet as far as possible underneath the anchor of the rings/TRX.

2. Let your arms straighten completely and then begin to pull your chest up to your hands, squeezing your shoulder blades together.

3. Slowly lower yourself back to the arms-extended position.

4. Repeat.

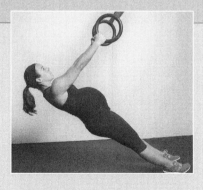
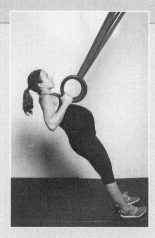

Pull Focus

Single-arm Dumbbell Back Row (Pull focus)

   1. Kneel on the bench by placing the knee and hand of your supporting arm on the bench. Position the foot of your opposite leg slightly back and to the side. Grasp the dumbbell from the floor.

   2. Pull the dumbbell up to the side until it makes contact with your ribs or until your upper arm is just beyond horizontal.

   3. Return until your arm is extended and your shoulder is stretched downward.

   4. Repeat and continue with your opposite arm.

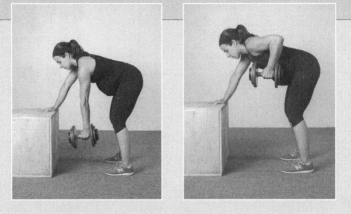

Single- or Double-arm Tubing Back Row (Pull focus)

   1. Secure tubing on a support. Grasp the tubing handle with one hand, allowing your shoulder to be pulled forward by the weight/tension.

   2. Pull the handle to the side of your torso while pulling your shoulder back, arching your spine, and pushing your chest forward.

   3. Return until your arm is extended and your shoulder is pulled forward.

   4. Repeat and continue with the opposite arm.

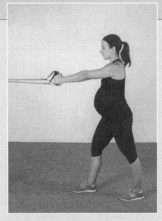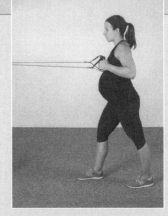

Push Focus

Barbell Push Jerk (Compound Movement and Push focus)

1. Stand holding the barbell with an overhand grip slightly wider than shoulder width.

2. Inhale and position your chest high with your torso tight. Keeping the pressure on your heels, dip your body by bending your knees and ankles slightly.

3. Explosively drive upward with your legs, driving the barbell up off your shoulders. Drop your body downward and split one foot forward and other backward as fast as possible while vigorously extending your arms overhead. The split position places your front shin vertical to the floor with your front foot flat on the floor. Your rear knee is slightly bent with your rear foot positioned on your toes. The bar should be positioned directly above your head at arms' length in line with your ears with your back straight.

4. Push up with both your legs. Position your feet side by side by bringing your front foot back partway and then your rear foot forward.

5. Lower the barbell to your shoulders. Then bend your knees slightly and lower the barbell to the midthigh position. Slowly lower the bar with a taut lower back and your trunk close to vertical.

6. Repeat.

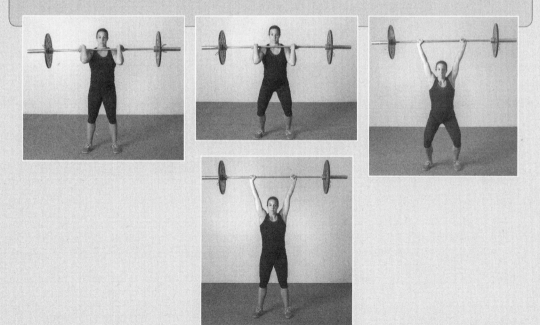

Note: The advanced athlete may unload (drop) the bar from the completed position. This technique may be practiced to reduce stress or fatigue involved in lowering the bar as prescribed. Use rubber weightlifting plates on a weightlifting platform if this unloading method is used (unless floor demolition is desired).

Push Focus

Bench or Physioball Alternating Bench Press (Push focus)

    1. Recline on a physioball so your upper back and neck are supported by the ball, and your hips are pressed up but are not supported by the ball. Hold one dumbbell in each hand.

    2. Lower one dumbbell to parallel to your chest and press out. While one arm is pressing, the other arm should be resting against your body.

    3. Repeat and alternate.

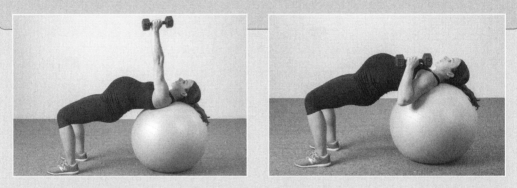

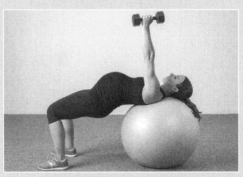

Donkey Calf Raises (Push focus)

1. Stand in a wide stance in a half squat position
2. Raise your heels by extending your ankles as high as possible, coming up onto your toes.
3. Lower your heels by bending your ankles until your calves are stretched.
4. Repeat.

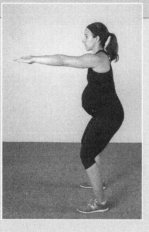 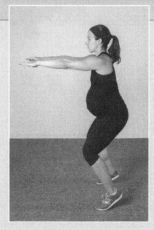

Push Focus

Dumbbell Chest Fly (Push focus)

1. Grasp two dumbbells. Lie supine on the bench or recline on a physioball so your upper back and neck are supported by the ball and your hips are pressed up but are not supported by the ball. Support the dumbbells above your chest with your arms fixed in a slightly bent position. Internally rotate your shoulders so your elbows point out to the sides.

2. Lower the dumbbells to your sides until your chest muscles are stretched with your elbows fixed in a slightly bent position.

3. Bring the dumbbells together in a hugging motion until the dumbbells are nearly together.

4. Repeat.

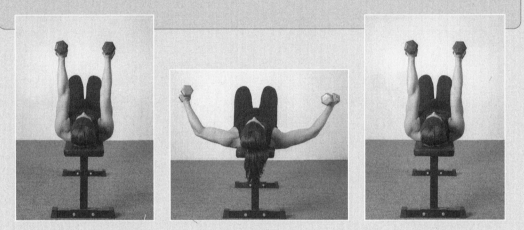

Dumbbell Single-arm Bicep Curl to Overhead Press (Push and Pull focus)

1. Position two dumbbells to your sides, palms facing in, arms straight.

2. With your elbows to your sides, raise one dumbbell and rotate your forearm until the forearm is vertical and your palm faces your shoulder.

3. With the dumbbell at shoulder level, press the weight straight up, finishing with the arm locked out and the bicep close to your ear.

4. Lower the weight back to your side and continue to alternate between sides.

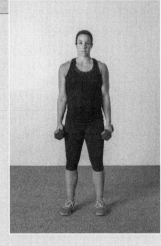 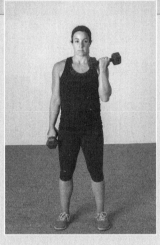 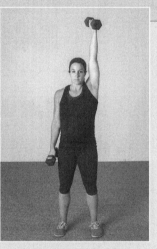

Push Focus

Dumbbell Skull Crusher (Push focus)

1. Lie on the bench with one dumbbell in each hand. Position the dumbbells over your shoulders with your arms extended.

2. Lower the dumbbells toward your forehead by bending your elbows.

3. Extend your arms and repeat.

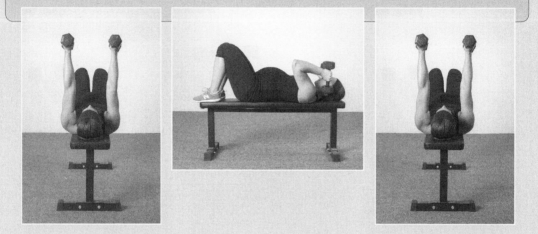

Dumbbell Push-Press (Push focus)

1. Begin with the dumbbells at shoulder level with your knuckles facing each other.

2. Dip your body by bending your knees, hips, and ankles slightly. Explosively drive upward with your legs, driving the dumbbells up off your shoulders, vigorously extending your arms overhead.

3. Return to your shoulders and repeat.

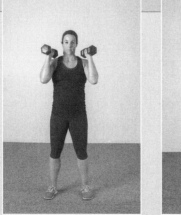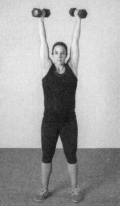

Dynamic Push-up (Push focus)

1. Lie prone on the floor with your hands slightly more than shoulder width apart.

2. Raise your body up off the floor by extending your arms with significant power and speed, keeping your body straight.

3. At the top of the push-up position, press harder into the ground, causing your hands to leave the ground.

4. Keeping your body straight, land with a soft bend in your elbows and lower your body to the floor by bending your arms.

5. Repeat.

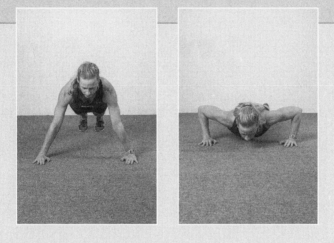

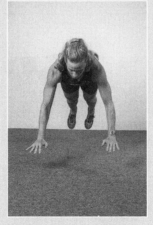

Push Focus

Handstand Push-ups (Push focus)

1. Stand facing a wall. Place hands on the floor and kick your lower body up to handstand position with your arms and legs straight. Maintain your balance with your lower body against the wall.

2. Lower your head until it touches the ground or pad(s), by bending your arms.

3. Push your body back up to your original position by extending your arms.

4. Repeat.

This can be modified by placing your feet on an incline bench in a pike position.

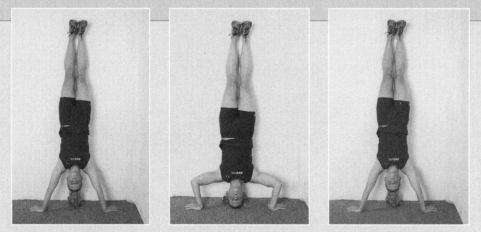

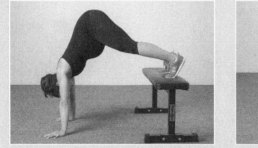
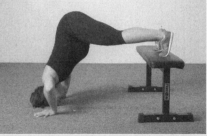

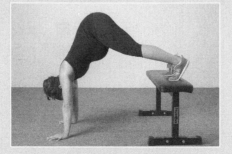

Inchworm Walkout (Push and Core focus)

1. From a standing position with your feet together or slightly apart, bend forward from your hips. Try to keep your legs straight (without locking your knees).

2. Put your hands on the ground and begin to walk your hands forward, away from your feet, until a full push-up position is reached.

3. Perform one full push-up.

4. Keeping your legs straight, walk your hands back to your feet.

5. Repeat.

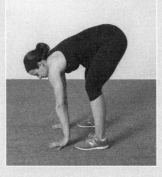

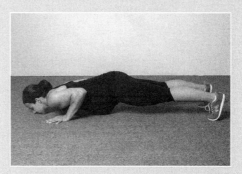

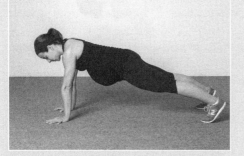

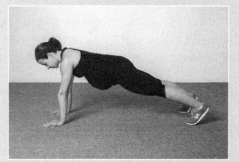

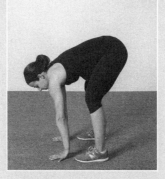

Push Focus

Medicine Ball Chattanooga Push-ups (Core and Push focus)
1. With a medicine ball under one hand, drop to a push-up while drawing your leg (medicine-ball side) out to the side of your body—pulling your knee up toward your elbow.
2. Switch the medicine ball and repeat on the other side.

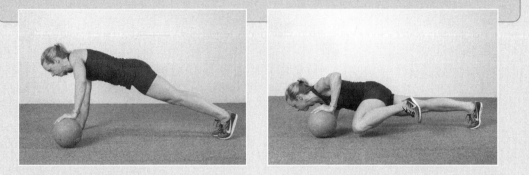

Overhead Press (Push focus)
1. Stand with feet shoulder width apart, holding a barbell or two dumbbells at shoulder level.
2. Press the weight straight up, finishing with your arms locked out and your bicep close to your ear.
3. Lower the weight and repeat.

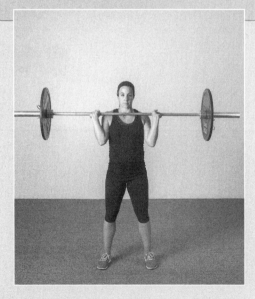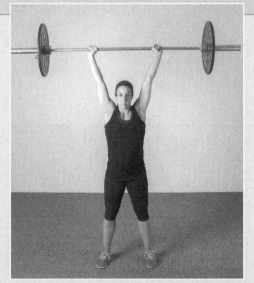

Physioball Single-arm Incline Chest Press (Push focus)

1. Recline on a physioball so your upper back and neck are supported by the ball, your hips are dropped so your lower back is close to or touching ball, but your glutes are still off the ground. Hold one dumbbell in each hand.

2. Raise the dumbbells over your shoulders and lower.

3. Press out one dumbbell at a time. Alternate your arms. While one arm is pressing, other arm should be in the locked-out position.

Physioball Single-arm, Single Dumbbell Unilateral Chest Press (Push focus)

1. Recline on a physioball so your upper back and neck are supported by the ball, and your hips are pressed up but are not supported by ball, while holding a dumbbell in each hand.

2. Lower the weight so it's parallel to your chest and press out.

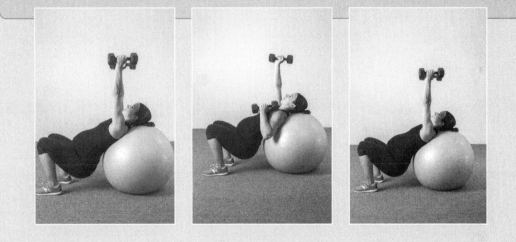

Push Focus

Physioball Walkout w/Push-up and Knee Tuck (Core and Push focus)

1. Start on your stomach on a physioball. Roll out forward so just your shins are on the ball.

2. Complete 1 push-up and then complete 1 knee tuck, pulling your thighs up into your chest.

3. Roll back until your chest is back on the ball.

4. Repeat.

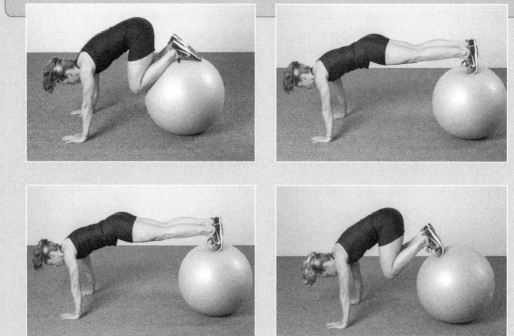

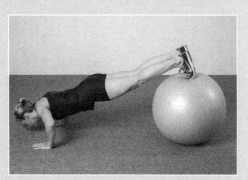 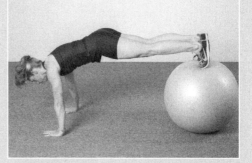

Push Focus

Pike Push-up (Push focus)

1. Kneel on a bench or box with your feet or knees slightly apart at the edge of the bench/box. Place your hands on the floor.

2. Raise your rear end high up with your arms, back, and knees straight. Adjust your feet so they are somewhat close to your hands while keeping your back and legs straight.

3. Lower your head by bending your arms.

4. Push your body back up to original position by extending your arms.

5. Repeat.

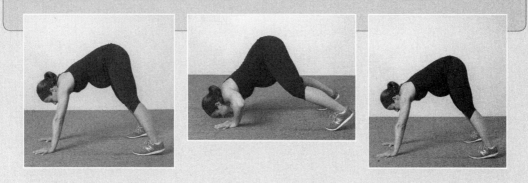

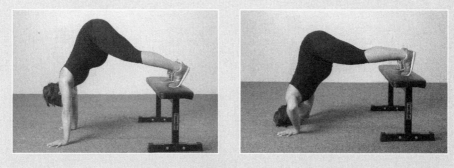

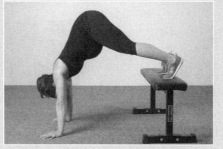

Push Focus

Push-Press (Push focus)

1. Grasp a barbell from the rack or clean a barbell from the floor with an overhand grip, slightly wider than shoulder width. Position the bar chest high with your torso tight. Retract your head back.

2. Dip your body by bending your knees, hips, and ankles slightly.

3. Explosively drive upward with your legs, driving the barbell up off your shoulders, vigorously extending your arms overhead.

4. Return to your shoulders and repeat.

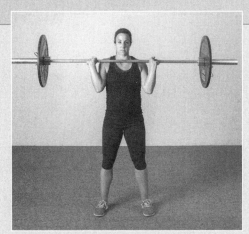

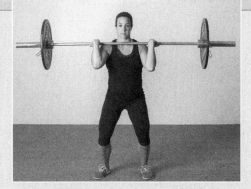

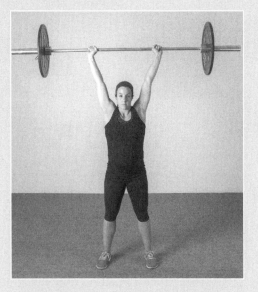

Push-up (Push focus)
1. Lie prone on the floor with your hands slightly wider than shoulder width.
2. Raise your body up off the floor by extending your arms with your body straight.
3. Keeping your body straight, lower your body to the floor by bending your arms.
4. Push your body up until your arms are extended.
5. Repeat.

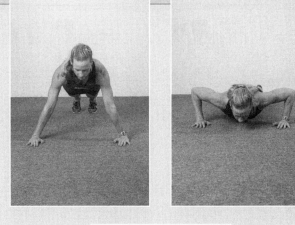

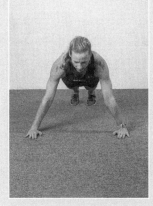

Push Focus

Unilateral Overhead Press (Push focus)

1. Stand with your feet shoulder width apart and hold a dumbbell in each hand at shoulder level.

2. One arm at a time, press straight up, finishing with the arm locked out and the bicep close to your ear.

3. Lower the extended arm and press up the other.

4. Repeat.

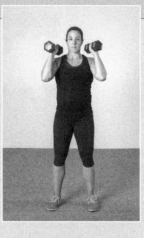 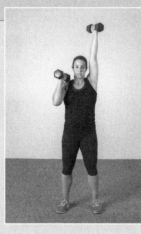

Wide-grip Push-up (Push focus)

1. Lie prone on the floor with your hands out as wide as you can comfortably place them.

2. Raise your body up off the floor by extending your arms with your body straight.

3. Keeping your body straight, lower your body to the floor by bending your arms.

4. Push your body up until your arms are extended.

5. Repeat.

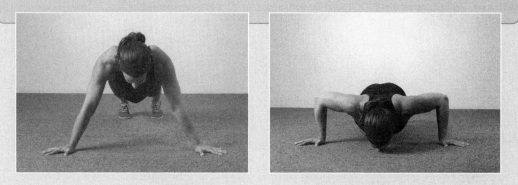

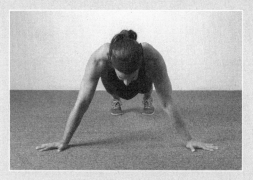

Push Focus

Yoga Push-up (Push and Core focus)
1. Start in a pike/Downward Facing Dog position.
2. Leading with your head, bend your arms and lower your body in a scooping motion to the floor, finishing in a Cobra position. Your body never touches/rests on the floor.
3. Reverse the motion to complete the move.

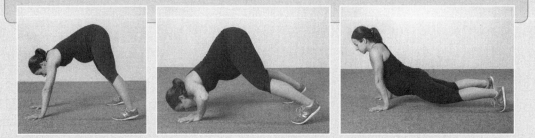

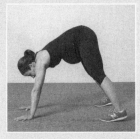 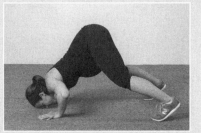

Squat Focus

Air/Body Weight Squat (Squat focus)

1. Stand with your feet shoulder width apart, your arms extended forward.

2. Squat down by bending your knees forward while allowing your hips to bend back behind, keeping your back straight and knees pointed in the same direction as your feet. Descend until your thighs are just past parallel to the floor.

3. Stand up by extending your knees and hips until your legs are straight.

4. Return and repeat.

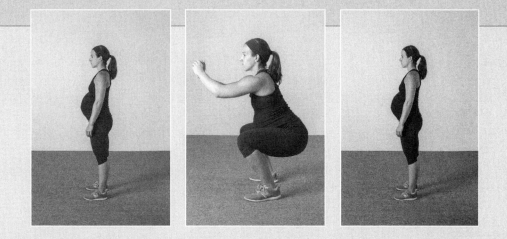

Ankle Band Air Squats (Squat focus)

1. Place an ankle band around both your ankles.

2. Stand with your feet shoulder-width apart and pull up ankle band around both legs to just below your kneecaps.

3. Perform a full-depth squat.

4. Repeat.

Squat Focus

Barbell Back Squat (Squat focus)
1. Position a barbell on the back of your shoulders and grasp the bar to the sides.
2. Bend your knees forward while allowing your hips to bend back behind, keeping your back straight and knees pointed in the same direction as your feet. Descend until your knees and hips are fully bent.
3. Extend your knees and hips until your legs are straight.
4. Return and repeat.

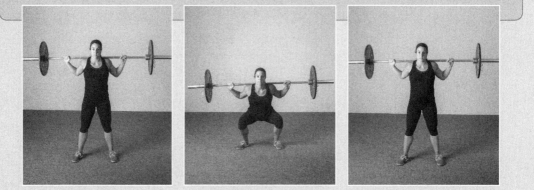

Barbell Front Squat (Squat focus)
1. Begin with a barbell resting on the front of your shoulders with your elbows flaring up and outward.
2. Bend your knees forward while allowing your hips to bend back behind, keeping your back straight and knees pointed in the same direction as your feet.
3. Descend until your thighs are just past parallel to the floor.
4. Extend knees and hips until legs are straight.
5. Return and repeat.

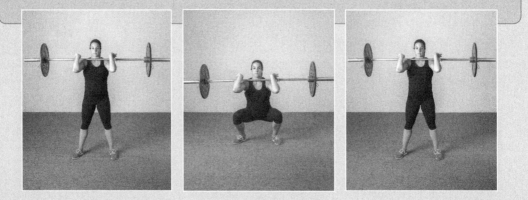

Barbell Split Squats (Squat focus)

1. Position a bar on the back of your shoulders. Position your feet far apart; one foot forward and other foot behind. Squat down by flexing the knee and hip of the front leg. Allow the heel of your rear foot to rise up while the knee of the rear leg bends slightly until it almost contacts the floor.

2. Return to your original standing position by extending the hip and knee of your forward leg.

3. Repeat. Continue with the opposite leg.

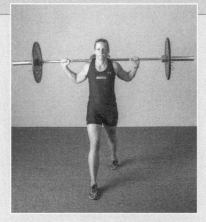
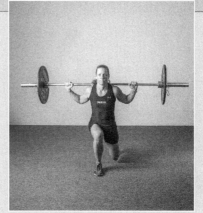
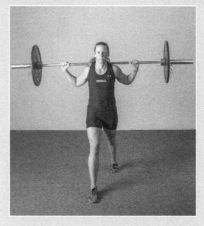

Squat Focus

Box Step-up (Squat focus)

1. Place the foot of the first leg on a box or bench.

2. Stand on the box/bench by extending the hip and knee of the first leg and place the foot of the second leg on the box/bench.

3. Step down with the second leg by flexing the hip and knee of the first leg.

4. Return to your original standing position by placing the foot of the first leg to the floor.

5. Repeat, alternating legs.

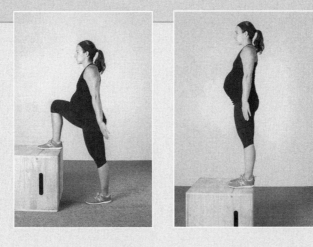

Squat Focus

Dumbbell Front Squat (Squat focus)

1. Begin with dumbbells at your shoulders so side of each dumbbell rests on top of each shoulder. Balance the dumbbells on your shoulder by holding onto the dumbbells with your elbows flaring outward.

2. Bend your knees forward while allowing your hips to bend back behind, keeping your back straight and your knees pointed in the same direction as your feet.

3. Descend until your thighs are just past parallel to the floor.

4. Extend your knees and hips until your legs are straight.

5. Return and repeat.

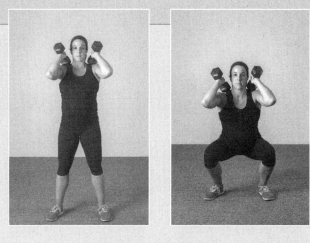

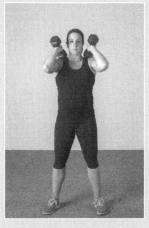

Squat Focus

Dumbbell Squat (Squat focus)
1. Stand with your feet shoulder width apart. Hold the dumbbells by your side.
2. Bend knees forward while allowing your hips to bend back behind, keeping your back straight and knees pointed in the same direction as your feet.
3. Descend until your knees and hips are fully bent.
4. Extend your knees and hips until your legs are straight.
5. Return and repeat.

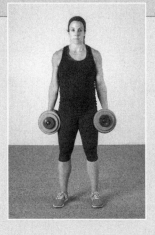 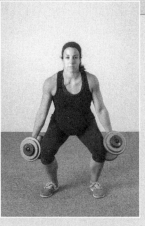 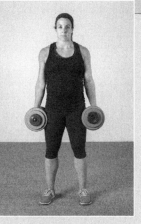

No-Touch Step-ups (Squat focus)
1. Stand on one foot on a box or bench with your other foot dangling over the side.
2. Bend your standing leg, drop the other foot toward the floor (try not to let the foot touch the floor), then raise it to the level of the box without allowing it to rest on the box.
3. Repeat, then move to other side.

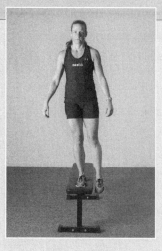
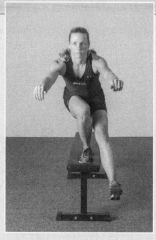

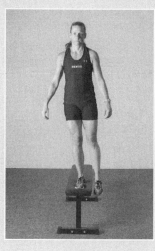

Squat Focus

Step-up to Reverse Lunge (with or without dumbbell) (Lunge focus)

1. Step up to a full upright position on a box.
2. Drop your nonstanding leg back to the lunge position. Try to touch your back knee to the floor.
3. Return both feet to the floor.
4. Step up next with your back leg (you will alternate feet).

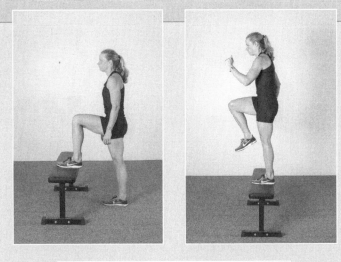

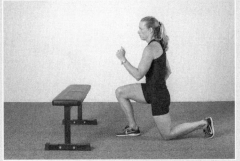

Note: If you are going to add weight, start light—5 to 8 pounds—and if you can still get through 3 sets of 20 reps without significant challenge, increase the weight. Choose a weight that creates challenge but as soon as your form and technique are compromised, decrease the weight.

Sumo Squat (Squat focus)

1. Stand with your feet a little more than shoulder width apart, a heavy dumbbell or kettlebell in both hands.
2. Lower the dumbbell to the floor, maintaining a straight back (look forward).
3. Raise to a standing position.
4. Repeat.

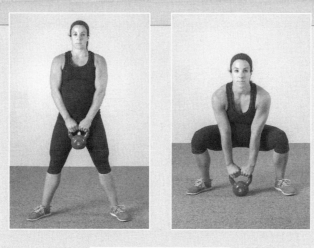

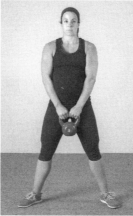

Index

Ovulation, 31, 32
Oxygen, 28, 62, 63, 151
  drop in, 55
  management, 115
  uptake of, 149

Pace, 114, 156
Pain, 31, 77, 141, 151
  back, 41, 63, 102, 135, 140
  calf, 123
  chest, 123
  low back, 89
  pelvic, 41, 103, 139
  toleration of, 66, 149, 151
Pain relief, 134, 135, 146
Parker, Candace, 68
PC muscle. *See* Pubococcygeus
  muscle
Pediatricians, looking for, 126
Pelvic floor, 118, 125, 129, 140, 150
  straining, 145
  strengthening, 89
  weight training and, 82
Pelvic girdle, 50, 63
Pelvic muscles, 49, 89
Pelvic prolapse, 147
Pelvic region, 68, 88, 100, 135, 137,
  147, 150
  overstressing, 73
  protecting, 92
Pelvic rest, 75
Pelvic tilt, 102, 150
Performance, 2, 69, 114, 115,
  123, 149
Perkins, Cooker, 43
Pertussis, increase in, 27
Physioball ABCs Plank (Core
  focus), described, 197
Physioball Double-leg Hamstring
  Curls (Pull focus), 142
  described, 216
Physioball Dumbbell Skull Crusher
  (Push focus), 142
Physioball Hamstring Curls (Pull
  focus), 95, 142
Physioball Single-arm DB Row
  (Pull focus), 48
Physioball Single-arm Incline
  Chest Press (Push focus), 142
  described, 231
Physioball Single-arm Row (Pull
  focus), described, 218

Physioball Single-arm, Single
  Dumbbell Unilateral Chest
  Press (Push focus), 35
  described, 231
Physioball Single-leg Hamstring
  Curls (Pull focus), described,
  217
Physioball Transfer (Core focus), 35
  described, 198
Physioball Unilateral Chest Fly
  (Push focus), 35
Physioball Walkout with Push-Up
  and Double-leg Knee Tuck
  (Core/Push focus), 71
  described, 199, 232
Physioballs, 21, 34, 47, 58, 70, 82,
  99, 101, 105, 119, 130, 140,
  142, 159
Pigeon stretch, 19
Pike Push-up (Push focus), 95
  described, 233, 234
Piriformis, 18, 19, 102
Placenta, 53, 86, 90, 100, 109,
  134, 140
  growth/efficiency of, 105
Placenta previa, 75, 123
Plank Single-arm Dumbbell
  Reverse Fly (Pull focus), 48
  described, 218
Plyo box, 20
Plyometrics, 103, 114, 118
  Box Jumps, 211
  Broad Jump, 212
  Squat Jumps, 212
Postdelivery workout, described,
  157–158
Posture, 92, 129
Preconception Strength Workout,
  described, 34–35
Preeclampsia, 33, 122
Premature delivery, exercise and,
  110
Premenstrual symptoms, 31, 79
Prenatal vitamins, 27, 32, 65
Presses, 154
  overhead, 148
  pike, 47
  shoulder, 47
  single-leg, 118
Progesterone, 31, 45, 50, 62
Progestogen, 82
Protein, 32, 54, 66, 86, 91

Pubococcygeus muscle (PC
  muscle), 89
Puffiness, 98–100
Pull focus, 9, 11, 161
  Bent Over, Straight-arm Tubing
    Pullbacks, 213
  Dumbbell Plank Rows, 213
  Dumbbell Single-arm Bicep
    Curl, 214
  Dumbbell Single-arm
    Bicep Curl to Overhead
    Press, 215
  Physioball Double-leg
    Hamstring Curls, 216
  Physioball Single-leg Hamstring
    Curls, 217
  Physioball Single-arm Row, 218
  Plank Single-arm Dumbbell
    Reverse Fly, 218
  Pull-up, 219
  Ring/TRS Rows, 219
  Single-arm Dumbbell Back
    Row, 220
  Single- or Double-Arm Tubing
    Back Row, 220
Pull-up bands, 22
Pull-up bars, 21, 58, 82, 95,
  106, 119
Pull-ups (Pull focus), 23
  described, 219
  in workout, 95, 130
Push focus, 9, 11, 161
  Barbell Push Jerk, 221
  Bench or Physioball Alternating
    Bench Press, 222
  Donkey Calf Raises, 223
  Dumbbell Chest Fly, 224
  Dumbbell Push-Press, 226
  Dumbbell Single-arm Bicep
    Curl to Overhead Press, 225
  Dumbbell Skull Crusher, 226
  Dynamic Push-up, 227
  Handstand Push-ups, 228
  Inchworm Walkout, 229
  Medicine Ball Chattanooga
    Push-ups, 230
  Overhead Press, 230
  Physioball Single-arm Incline
    Chest Press, 231
  Physioball Single-arm, Single
    Dumbbell Unilateral Chest
    Press, 231